DR. EARL MINDELL'S

WHAT YOU SHOULD KNOW ABOUT

Herbs, Supplements,
Trace Minerals,
and
Homeopathic Remedies

EARL L. MINDELL, R.PH., PH.D.
with VIRGINIA L. HOPKINS

ACKNOWLEDGMENTS

We would like to thank Maria Gordon, Larry Johns, and Kim Shepherd for their invaluable assistance.

This edition published by Barnes & Noble, Inc., by arrangement with Keats Publishing, a division of NTC/Contemporary Publishing Group, Inc. 4255 West Touhy Avenue, Lincolnwood, Illinois 60646-1975 U.S.A.

2000 Barnes & Noble Books

ISBN: 0-7607-2052-5

Printed and bound in the United States of America

DHD 00 01 02 M 9 8 7 6 5 4 3 2 1

CONTENTS

Herbs for Your Health

Creating Your Personal Vitamin Plan

Trace Minerals

Homeopathic Remedies 257

Dr. Earl Mindell's

What You Should Know About Herbs for Your Health

PART I
Herbs, Folklore and Pharmacy

Herbs, the Original Medicines

Can you imagine a world without bottles of aspirin and antibiotics? How would you feel if your doctor had no drugs to prescribe for serious illnesses? This was the world of our not-so-distant ancestors and, what's more, it still exists today in Third World countries. Yet it is precisely this primitive world that we owe for all the benefits of modern medicine we enjoy.

The pharmaceutical industry has learned to harness the power of many natural substances, producing synthetic versions which have become our prescription and over-the-counter drugs. These have brought undoubted advances, but often at the cost of debilitating side effects and complications.

Meanwhile, more and more scientific research is serving to remind us of nature's own safer, gentler packages of healing power which lie behind so many of today's drugs. The truth is that remedies like Grandma's elderberry wine and the Chickasaw Indians' infusion of willow root are scientifically proven! As more and more natural remedies are tested and refined, the apparent need for expensive drugs with dangerous side effects declines. Science is showing real medical advances are in store as we learn to combine old wisdom with new.

WHAT IS AN HERB?

Any plant with medicinal properties is called an herb. Of course, herbs can also be plants used as food, or in cosmetics, or for seasoning or flavoring. Herbs used to treat physical conditions are plants that in some way demonstrate a healing effect.

Herbs are the main source of medicine for the primary care needs of possibly 80 percent of the world's population. This was the World Health Organization's estimate in 1985. In the U.S. herbs have been overtaken by manufactured drugs only in the past 60 years. Until World War II, the *U.S. Pharmacopoeia*, the listing of officially accepted medicines, included herbal preparations. Even today, nearly 40 percent of prescribed drugs dispensed in the U.S. are either based on or are synthesized versions of natural substances. In a way, herbs could be said to be the forgotten or hidden healing element of modern medicine.

CHAPTER 1

The Ancient Tradition of Herbal Medicines

Chrysanthemum as an antibiotic? It's true, and, would you believe it, used by chimpanzees! Zoologists in Africa have seen one species regularly dosing themselves with this potent plant. All of us have seen sick cats and dogs eating grass. Imagine human intelligence and curiosity combined with instinct, and it's easy to see how prehistoric cultures must have developed considerable knowledge of the medicinal properties of the plants around them.

We no longer have to chew on buckthorn and discover its purgative effects by accident! Someone long ago ate lobelia flowers and ended up with their head over an ancient toilet. It is modern science that labels these things as laxatives and emetics, but it was wise, observant people of the past who discovered them and realized that their actions could relieve illness. Indeed, the remains of plants known as herbal remedies such as bramble, crab apple, orache (a spinach-like weed) and wild service tree have been found in the pots and waste pits of Neolithic villages in England and Switzerland. The recording of such remedies began as civilization advanced, allowing us to trace fascinating herbal treatments from every culture far back into history.

Traditional herbal medicine in India, called Ayurveda, goes back more than 5,000 years. As far back as 3,000 B.C., official schools of herbalism existed in Egypt, teaching about plants like garlic, mint, and coriander. Cleopatra is said to have used cucumber to preserve her skin and the *Ebers Papryus*, written about 1,500 B.C., recommends applying a moldy piece of bread to open wounds, thousands of years before Alexander Fleming developed penicillin from the very same mold.

The Chinese were using oil from hydnocarpus trees to treat leprosy as early as 2,500 B.C. Centuries later came the *Shen Nong Ben Cao Jing*, China's first true herbal, describing more than 350 plants used for medicinal purposes. The Chinese were also using ephedrine, our over-the-counter cold medication, in the form of the shrub ma huang, over two thousand years ago.

Although a religious work, the Bible is another rich source of herbal references from cinnamon to myrrh, with mandrakes even serving as aphrodisiacs in the Genesis story of Jacob's wives, Leah and Rachel.

Early European settlers in America were amazed at and often thankful for the range of medicinal applications for herbs used by the Indians for needs from headaches to heart conditions. Tribes such as the Iroquois and Mohegans treated colds and fevers with tea made from the boneset plant. Wormwood was a bronchitis and cold remedy used by Indians as far apart as New Mexico and British Columbia. Thompson Indians would stuff their nostrils with wormwood leaves to relieve nasal congestion and when burying decaying corpses! As America was settled, remedies were exchanged. Europeans for example learned of soothing witch hazel ointment from the North Americans, and Indians learned to use dandelion remedies for conditions like heartburn as the plant was introduced to their country.

Some American Indian, and European, and Eastern remedies were often selected in a similar manner, referred to as the Doctrine of Signatures. A plant would be used to treat a condition of a body part which it resembled. Liverleaf, with liver-shaped leaves, for example, was used to treat liver disorders. Science has even proven links for plants such as red bloodroot as a "blood purifier" and the yellowish goldenseal root for the treatment of jaundice.

European herbal remedies, passed down through village wise women, sold by wandering herbalists, and often copied by monks from ancient Greek and Roman writings, were used by royalty and peasants alike. Queen Elizabeth I is said to have favored meadowsweet, used to treat flu, fever and arthritis. From Roman times, lavender was known to promote relaxation, while chervil was recommended as a stimulant— one that also reportedly cured hiccups if you ate the whole plant! Arabs, too, used Greek and Roman texts, elaborating on remedies with often highly sweetened preparations and exotic spices. Herbs such as ginger and cardamom were believed to prevent illness.

The herbals of 16th and 17th century Europe make colorful reading today. Would you swallow sumac powder if you were advised that it had "great efficacy in strengthening the stomach and bowels?" Would you wash "pestiferous sores" with wild succory? How about calamint to kill "all manner of worms in the body"? We might smile and raise our eyebrows at some of these ancient herbal treatments, but science today is telling us loud and clear that many a plant prescription makes as much, if not more sense, than a modern drug equivalent.

CHAPTER 2

From Folklore to Pharmaceutical

Observation, trial and error, and faith seem to have been key to the practice of early Western herbalism. It came with no real system or rules until the second century A.D. and a Greek called Galen, physician to a Roman Emperor. Galen's Herbal marked the beginning of a trend separating the professional physician from the traditional healer. Influenced by Galen and his rigid rules, medicine began to be taught in Europe as a superior art favoring exotic medicines with aggressive treatments such as bloodletting and purging.

Following the failure of this style of doctoring to help in the Black Plague of 1348 and again with outbreaks of syphilis, Galenic practice began to be challenged in Europe in the 16th and 17th centuries. Herbalists such as the famous Englishman, Nicholas Culpeper, helped expose the false mystery and monopoly of "official" medicine and brought simple, garden-grown remedies back to popularity. Brutal attempts at dramatic cures with practices like medical bleeding eventually died out, but not before George Washington was bled to death in 1797 during treatment for a sore throat.

The Swiss physician and alchemist, Paracelsus, who developed laudanum, also influenced the return to the idea that medicines were found by searching for cures held by plants. He even predicted that pharmacologically "active principles" would be found in herbs. Ironically, it may have been the observation of just such active compounds in the plant, digitalis, that set orthodox medicine on the path of the synthetic drugs that came to replace herbs. In 1785, the English doctor William Withering detailed the biological effects and recommended doses of the plant digitalis. His work led eventually to the discovery of the modern heart stimulants digoxin and digitoxin.

Digitalis probably helped standard physicians continue to focus on the idea of the quick fix, in demand, too, of course, by the public. Although figures like Thomas Jefferson still cultivated herbs in kitchen gardens, 18th century chemists worked hard in laboratories to isolate and synthesize active ingredients and bypass the plants themselves. In this way, the modern pharmaceutical industry was born.

In a move to help companies recover the costs of research and development of synthetic substances, the American government passed a patent medicine law in the late 1800s. This gave companies the exclusive 17-year rights to sell patented drugs. Unfortunately, it also gave them an incentive to discredit the use of natural remedies in order to maximize profits from synthetic ones. Formation of the Federal Drug Administration (FDA) made the situation even worse for natural remedies. There is no incentive at all to gain FDA approval for an herbal medicine when it takes 10 to 18 years and costs millions of dollars with no patent protection at the end of it all!

In countries like France and Germany, however, the system for approval of medicines is different, and many natural medications are sold over-the-counter and prescribed. No health claims can be made in America for herbal remedies, which must be sold as foods or supplements. Thanks also to the American Medical Association (AMA) support and huge marketing campaigns, it's not surprising that synthetic drugs have dominated American medical teaching and treatment since the 1950s. However, surveys show the majority of Americans take supplements of some sort, and increasing numbers of physicians are beginning to integrate modern and traditional practices. The Program in Integrative Medicine at the University of Arizona, for example, is part of a new teaching trend which integrates alternative medicine with mainstream medicine. The future could take a very different path.

CHAPTER 3

Natural or Synthetic? A Question of Balance

Heart attack? Broken leg? Life-threatening infection? Western emergency treatment is the proven choice. But it's estimated that emergencies make up only about 20 percent of conditions treated by doctors. Viral infections, degenerative diseases, cancers, auto-immune diseases and other illnesses make up the other 80 percent. With the majority of illnesses, the focus of modern medicine has been the relief of symptoms. The aim with herbal remedies, on the other hand, is the restoration of health by treating the underlying cause.

Early herbalists regarded themselves as "nature's servants" and respected the body's natural efforts to return to wellness. Western pharmaceutical companies act more like nature's masters, attempting to manipulate biochemical functions in isolation from each other. The drugs they produce are concentrated versions of compounds recognized by the cells of our bodies. This is why they achieve their often fast and dramatic effects. However, to make an effective substance patentable, drug companies must add molecules that make the drug synthetic, or not found in nature. These extra molecules create additional biological reactions as they are processed—reactions we call side effects.

In contrast, herbal remedies package their active chemicals with beneficial substances that ameliorate side effects. This packaging can make the active compound more easily absorbed, as with the uptake of iron aided by the vitamin C in plants like watercress and rose hips. Other chemical combinations in herbs seem to be built-in safety measures. Ephedrine, isolated from the ma huang plant, was once prescribed for asthma, but produced the side effect of dangerously high blood pressure levels. The whole plant has been used for thousands of years with no harmful results. The difference? Six related chemicals in the herb itself, one of which actually lowers blood pressure and reduces heart rate. Aspirin can relieve pain and fever, but may cause stomach bleeding. Its natural derivative, white willow bark, is without this unwanted effect.

Scientific analysis bears out the observation that the effects of chemicals in plants often have parallel effects in humans. Plants such as cranberries contain substances which help to preserve them by killing bacteria. The same substances have similar effects in our bodies. This sort of phenomenon is not surprising, as every living thing is made of the same basic constituents such as proteins and sugars, and since they have all evolved from the same origins.

Medicinal plants also echo the body's own life-maintaining system of checks and balances. Ginseng, for instance, contains hormone-like substances called saponins. Some have a sedative effect, others are stimulating. The body, then, will naturally utilize the different saponins according to its needs. Ginseng, as a result, is a body stabilizer, increasing the ability of the body to withstand stress. Hawthorn berries work on blood pressure in the same way with a mixture of compounds which either raise or lower blood pressure. Expert herbalists are able to extend this process by creating remedies which are a combination of plants with a selected balance of effects.

Western medicine's pill-popping habits have led to passive, often fearful, but unquestioning patients who do not expect to take much part in their own recovery. Herbal medicine differs in that it demands a review of the body's overall condition as well as specific symptoms. Herbs themselves, and the way they are used, are more likely than synthetic drugs to address underlying conditions. The care, cultivation and mixing of herbs also brings respect for and conservation of natural resources.

While the advances brought about by modern medicine are obvious, Western levels of conditions like heart disease, hypertension and cancer are appallingly high. Complications from prescription drugs result in 40 percent of hospitalizations and cause 20,000 to 30,000 deaths every year in the United States. Yet, this is an age where a balance can be struck. Powerful, short-term treatment with synthetic drugs is a proven option. Gentle, safe, longer-term herbal medications deserve a role alongside as nature's complete pharmacy, evolved in natural harmony with the human body.

SCIENCE PROVES THE VALUE OF HERBS

Slaves building the Egyptian pyramids once went on strike over their rations of garlic! Today they would have scientific proof of its benefits—so much of it that even the U.S. medical establishment cannot falsely claim that none exists. Recent years have produced 2,000 studies on garlic by researchers all over the world. It has been shown to be antimicrobial, antibiotic, antiviral, antiparasitic, anticancer and an immune booster. Substances found in garlic include antioxidants, smooth muscle relaxants and four powerful anti-clotting agents. Studies have shown how these substances help garlic prevent and relieve heart disease. Garlic also inhibits an enzyme which generates an inflammatory chemical, explaining claims for its use with asthma.

Another ancient remedy proven effective by science is chamomile, used for centuries in Europe against infections and aches. Modern analysis shows it is an antispasmodic in the bowel and stomach with a sedative effect on the central nervous system. It also contains anti-inflammatories which contribute to its usefulness in ointments and lotions.

A North American remedy now validated scientifically is the purple coneflower, echinacea. This plant was used medicinally by native Indians more than any other plant. Echinacea treatments existed for wounds, burns, abscesses, insect bites, snake bites, toothache, joint pains and infections. Chemical analysis of echinacea reveals a fascinating combination of substances, including some with antiviral and anticancer properties and others which regenerate tissue. Interestingly, the antibiotic properties of echinacea are mild. Instead, scientists have found it is the strong immune enhancing activity of echinacea compounds which lie behind its power against internal and external bacterial infections.

A popular folk remedy for colds and flu, elderberry, has high concentrations of bioflavonoids. These could account for the recently proven ability of elderberry extract to kill flu viruses. A recent double-blind study using the commercial elderberry extract Sambucol more than halved the recovery time for sufferers of flu compared to subjects given placebos. As a winter tonic, elderberry is now official.

Chemicals called PCOs are the main effective agents in another berry, the bilberry or European blueberry. Bilberry jam was eaten to improve the night vision of

World War II pilots. Bilberry extract has indeed been shown to improve the ability of the eyes to adapt from dark to light. It also prevents and retard cataracts and ulcers and lowers blood sugar, so proving its folk use in the treatment of diagnosis. What's more, its smooth muscle relaxing effects have been demonstrated in experiments, showing exactly why it became a treatment for vascular disorders.

Another excellent example of an herb which shines under the spotlight of modern science is ginger. Used for thousands of years in China, ginger is shown to be high in antioxidants, to inhibit inflammation triggers and blood clotting agents, to kill bacteria and reduce cholesterol levels. Animal studies confirm ginger's historic use in warming the body and treating ulcers.

Experiments also show important differences in the composition of dry and raw ginger. They serve, too, to show why the effects of herbs like garlic and licorice change depending on their form. The standards of modern analysis and testing producing these kinds of observations give added reassurance to users of herbal remedies. They form a technological supplement to the huge volume of historical evidence for the efficacy of herbs. And they often stem, ironically, from the research used to produce synthetic drugs! Perhaps the pendulum is due now to rest between traditional herbal and modern medicines.

THE RACE FOR MODERN HERBAL DISCOVERIES IS ON

Did you know a major ingredient of birth control pills comes from wild yam or that quinine, the malaria drug, is derived from the Peruvian "fever tree," the cinchona? A surprising amount of the world's harvest goes to help produce the drugs of our time. Unhappily, the potential harvest has been dwindling at an amazing rate as land is cleared or developed. Experts like Tom Eisner, Schurman Professor of Biology at Cornell, point out that only about 2 percent of known plant species have been analyzed thoroughly for their pharmacological effects. Even worse, botanists estimate that millions of plants have still to be named and many have already been lost forever to environmental destruction. Only recently, logging operations in Pacific northwest forests burned Pacific yew as slash. Then came the discovery of the anti-cancer drug, taxol, in, yes, the bark of the Pacific yew tree. There is no doubt that many effective compounds must have already been lost as unknown species have been wiped out.

Naturalists and scientists have been spurred to work together to fully investigate the wealth of species already collected and to campaign for environmental preservation measures. The profit motive actually brings the cooperation of drug companies, too, which continually search for new plant drugs to synthesize. The payoff can be big, in medical and money terms, with finds like the rosy periwinkle, which has produced two anticancer drugs used successfully to treat childhood leukemias and Hodgkin's disease. This was an accidental spin-off of a drug company's search for antidiabetic agents. Drugs like the fungus-derived cyclosporin, an immune suppressant used in organ transplants, and ivermectin, a parasitic worm killer, have also been uncovered relatively recently.

Only a small percentage of known plants has already yielded tremendous medical benefit. It's simply common sense to continue the research and investigation of the depleted stocks of laboratory Earth while ensuring, too, that we don't burn down the laboratory itself.

MEDICINAL HERBS IN OTHER CULTURES

Because herbs are the main form of medicine for most
cultures of the world, and pharmaceutical drugs are,
relatively speaking, much more expensive and cause
thousands of deaths every year, the World Health Organization is studying and promoting herbal medicines. Natural medicines have come into their own as
inexpensive, safe and effective treatments easily acces-
sible to their native users. There is a real opportunity
for developing cultures to integrate natural remedies
with the benefits of modern medicine and none of
the penalties.

China, with its established and ancient herbal tradition, has been integrating positive aspects of Western
medicine faster than natural remedies have been re-
vived in the West. A revival is happening, however,
and on an international scale. Many physicians from
India also train in the U.S. and Europe, blending Ayurvedic and Western medicine in their practices. Scientific research has spurred fresh interest, seeing sales
of herbal products pass $4 billion in Germany alone,
and higher figures in Japan.

Use of herbal remedies as standard medicines in
different countries probably never dipped as low as
they did in the U.S. with its restrictive FDA regula-
tions. Herbal medicines and modern drugs face the
same legal tests in Germany, and insurance reimburses
the costs of herbal remedies sold in pharmacies when
they are prescribed by a doctor. One of the top three
most widely prescribed drugs in both Germany and
France is ginkgo biloba, used to treat certain vascular
disorders. In the U.S., gingko biloba can only be sold
as a food supplement. German physicians might also
prescribe the herb valerian to treat mild anxiety. Homeopathic remedies are very widely prescribed in
France. In Great Britain, natural remedies have always

sat side by side with synthetic remedies on drug store shelves.

Around the world, cultural gravity seems to be working to pull Western medicine back down to its herbal roots. The weight of scientific evidence only adds to the pull, with the message that stronger links with nature are good medicine everywhere on Earth.

PART II
A Guide to My Favorite
Healing Herbs

CHAPTER 4

How to Use the Healing Herbs

As modern technology becomes increasingly sophisticated, we are discovering more and more about just how complex plant ingredients are. We used to believe that beta-carotene was the only useful vitamin in a carrot. Now we know that in a raw carrot there are hundreds of carotenoids, of which beta-carotene is only one. In addition, a raw carrot is packed with vitamins, minerals, sugars, enzymes, fibers, and dozens of other substances we don't fully understand yet.

Think of celery and lettuce. For years we were told they had no nutritional value. Now we know that if you eat six stalks of celery a day your blood pressure will almost certainly drop. Lettuce contains ingredients that can make you sleepy. It's not that these vegetables had no nutritional value, it's just that until recently, our technology and science weren't advanced enough to understand them!

Any healing herb or medicinal plant is a veritable chemistry lab of ingredients with specific biochemical actions and reactions in the human body. These include volatile oils which give plants their aroma, sterols which have similarities to our own steroid hormones, saponins which have "soapy" qualities, and alkaloids, which are often poisonous to the liver but which sometimes have profound healing properties.

Each healing herb listed here has specific effects on the body, based on its chemical makeup. The chemicals that have the strongest effects on the tissues and organs of the body are called *active principles*. Plants rich in active principles are the most valuable as medicines. It is the active principles in plants that the pharmaceutical companies attempt to isolate, patent and turn into pharmaceutical drugs. But what we have found, over and over again, is that once an active principle is isolated from the other ingredients in a plant, it has side effects. Somehow in the miraculous wisdom of nature, a whole herb prepared and taken properly has very few if any, side effects. The synergy or combination of ingredients working together in a plant brings a balance to it as a medicine that makes herbal medicine gentle and yet still effective.

While herbal medicines are more gentle than pharmaceutical drugs, don't be fooled into thinking that herbs can be used carelessly. A wide range of potency and toxicity exists among the healing herbs. Women who are pregnant or nursing, and anyone with a serious chronic illness such as diabetes or heart disease, should carefully research an herb, or consult with a health care professional familiar with herbs, before using it.

For example, angelica can be a wonderful herb for indigestion, and for inducing sweating in a cold. But because it increases circulation, it can also promote menstruation, so it shouldn't be used by pregnant women. Another active principle in angelica can cause it to increase the amount of sugar in the blood, so it shouldn't be used by diabetics without supervision.

Your doctor is unlikely to encourage you to use herbal medicine. He or she was told in medical school that herbs were unscientific, superstitious folklore. Doctors are trained that their job is to diagnose a disease and then find a drug to prescribe for the symptoms of the disease. While I know that you're going to get a negative response ranging from condescen-

sion to dire warnings if you tell your doctor you're
taking herbs, I encourage you not to self-treat yourself
with herbs if you have a serious or chronic condition.
Seek out a doctor who uses natural medicines, or find
a naturopathic doctor. Many chiropractors are also
skilled in the use of natural medicines.

IF YOU'RE TAKING OTHER MEDICATIONS

I want you to be aware that mixing herbs with pharmaceutical drugs can cause the drug to overreact or un-
derreact. For example, ephedra may help dry up your
sinuses, but it also can raise blood pressure and increase heart rate, which could be dangerous for someone taking a heart drug. In another example,
echinacea won't interfere with an antibiotic, but because it stimulates the immune system, it could interfere with an immunosuppressive drug such as a
cortisone.

On the other side of the coin, taking herbs that
support your body can help alleviate the side effects
of a prescription drug. For example, if you're taking
acetaminophen (Tylenol), which is very hard on the
liver, taking milk thistle (silymarin) will help support
your liver.

I realize you can't possibly figure out all the possible
interactions of drugs, foods and herbs, but I want you
to be aware that herbs do have specific biochemical
actions in the body and use caution. My best advice
to you is to use common sense and moderation, and
follow the proper dosage instructions.

As a pharmacist I am well aware that no two people
respond to a medicine in the same way. Each person's
biochemistry is unique. Your weight, age, sex, how
much you exercise, your diet, and whether you use
drugs such as alcohol and caffeine, will all affect how
you respond to an herbal medicine.

If you try an herb and feel worse, stop taking it. If you try an herb and nothing happens, try half again to twice as much. If there is still no result, this probably isn't the herb for you. (Some herbs take 2-4 weeks to affect the system in a noticeable way. Again, do your research.)

IF YOU'RE PREGNANT

When you're pregnant you want to avoid putting anything in your body that would disrupt or interfere with the growth of the fetus. Please don't take herbs of any kind if you're pregnant without checking first with an experienced health professional familiar with herbs. There are a few herbs, such as raspberry leaf, which can be beneficial to take when you're pregnant, and there are specific herbs to help with labor and to start breast milk flowing. However, these should only be used with an experienced professional.

DO YOUR RESEARCH

Before taking any herb, do your homework. That could be as simple as referring to this book, or it could mean buying a more detailed herb book and doing some in-depth research. Don't use an herb long-term without thoroughly checking it out. Powerful herbs such as ephedra should never be used for more than a week or two at a time.

CHAPTER 5

My Top Twenty-Nine Healing Herbs

ARNICA (Arnica montana)

Also commonly called leopard's bane, arnica is a perennial herb found singly or in small clusters in mountainous regions. Its bright yellow, daisy-like flower heads bloom around July.

The volatile oils from the dried flower heads of European arnica have been used since the 11th century largely as a topical pain reliever and as an application to treat bruises and sprains. The Catawba Indians used a tea of arnica root resins for treating back pains. In old Russia, the herb was used internally to reduce cholesterol, promote production of bile, stimulate the nervous system, stop bleeding and to strengthen the heart.

Externally, the classic use of arnica is for muscle, joint or cartilage pain which is generally aggravated by movement and alleviated by rest. Typically, arnica is rubbed on the skin to soothe and heal bruises, sprains, hyperextensions, wounds, irritations and to provide relief due to muscle spasm, arthritis or bursitis. Placed on the stomach, a compress containing arnica can relieve abdominal pains. Applied as a salve, arnica is also good for chapped lips, irritated nostrils and acne. Only a highly diluted form of arnica should be used when the surface of the skin is broken. Too strong a concentration can cause blistering. There are a wide variety of arnica creams and salves available at your health food store.

Internally, tinctures of arnica are used for mental and physical shock, pain and swelling, concussion, fractured bones, sprains, dental extractions and headache. Some doctors have used the herb for internal bleeding, obstinate sore throat and inflammation of the mouth. Arnica should never be used internally without medical direction because an overdose can be fatal.

Arnica works by stimulating activity of white blood cells (macrophages) that perform much of the digestion of congested blood and by dispersing trapped, disorganized fluids from banged, bumped and bruised tissues, muscles and joints.

ALOE VERA (Aloe barbadensis)

It's common to see a spiky house plant with thick, rubbery, tapering green leaves edged with spiny teeth in a pot sitting around homes. Those wise to the ways of herbal healing keep it in the kitchen. The plant is aloe vera, or lily of the desert, and for most people it is there waiting to exude a mucilaginous sap when broken as first aid to quickly spread over a burn to relieve pain and prevent blisters. However, the skin-healing properties of aloe are not limited to burns.

In Africa, prior to hunting, natives rub the gel of the aloe over their bodies to remove the human scent. Women all over the world apply aloe gel on their skin to keep it supple and to clear blemishes. Greek history records the use of aloe as a healing herb for wounds 2,000 years ago. Legend has it Cleopatra massaged the gel into her skin every day. Napoleon's wife, Josephine, is said to have used a lotion of aloe and milk for her complexion.

In Ayurvedic medicine, aloe gel is a tonic for the female reproductive system. At one time people rubbed it into their scalps, believing it prevented hair loss. The gel is used to treat ulcers, ring worms, shingles, and to repel insects.

Aloe reportedly helps to clear pimples and acne. Dermatologists have also had success treating oily skin, dandruff, and psoriasis. By applying aloe to their nipples, nursing mothers can begin to reduce the supply of milk, thereby serving as an aid to weaning. And, aloe has been found to aid in the treatment of frostbite.

The medicinal properties of aloe have now been scientifically substantiated. Research documents its healing effect of all kinds of burns and the itch caused by poison ivy and oak. Additional studies have confirmed the anesthetic, antibacterial, and tissue restorative properties of this remarkable herb. The gel does indeed heal burns from the sun or a hot pan, and when not severe, regenerates tissue without scarring.

Aloe is believed to improve wound healing by increasing the availability of oxygen and by increasing the synthesis and strength of collagen and tissue.

BILBERRY (Vaccinium myrtillus)

The bilberry, or European blueberry, is a perennial shrub that grows in meadows and woods in Europe. Only the blue-black berries of the plant are used. These differ from the American blueberry in that the meat of the bilberry fruit is blue-black throughout.

Bilberry has long been a folk remedy for poor vision and "night blindness." During World War II, British Royal Air Force pilots reported improved vision on night bombing raids after eating bilberry jam.

Clinical tests confirm that bilberry given orally to humans not only improves visual accuracy in healthy people, but also helps those with eye diseases such as pigmentosa, retinitis, glaucoma and myopia. Components in the herb work specifically to improve vision by improving microcirculation and speeding the regeneration of retinal purple, a substance required for good eyesight.

Bilberry extract has been widely used in connection with vascular, or blood vessel disorders. Specific studies reveal a positive effect in the treatment of varicose veins, thrombosis and angina. The active components of bilberries are its flavonoids, which serve to prevent capillary fragility, inhibit platelet aggregation and stimulate the release of vasodilators, substances which open up blood vessels and improve the flow of blood, thus increasing the level of oxygen in tissues.

Recent research has also indicated that bilberry extract possesses significant preventive and curative anti-ulcer properties, attributed to the strengthening of the defensive barriers of the digestive system.

CALENDULA (Calendula officinalis)

A featured plant in many ornamental gardens, calendula or pot marigold, is a hardy, many-branched annual, almost entirely covered with fine hairs. The yellow-to-deep orange flowers ray out from a central head and close up at night.

Ancient Romans named this plant, noting that the flowers were in bloom on the first day, or calends, of every month. They also grew calendulas to treat scorpion bites. In early use, the herb was also used to treat headaches, fevers and toothaches. A 16th century concoction which called for the use of calendula was thought to enable one to see fairies.

Calendula came to America with settlers from Europe and was used during the Civil War to help stop bleeding and promote the healing of wounds.

Medically, calendula flower tinctures have been recommended in the treatment of a wide variety of ailments, including fever, cramps, flu, and stomach aches. Others apply calendula-based remedies to external sores, cuts, bruises, burns and rashes. Calendula flowers are said to relieve the pain of bee stings. And when applied directly to the ear, calendula oil can reduce earache pain. Mothers find it works well as a solution for diaper rash. Calendula and arnica are often combined in commercial skin ointments for burns and bruises.

Calendula tea can be used as an eye wash for sore, reddened eyes. As a cosmetic, calendula brings out highlights in blond and brunette hair, and is found in herbal bath mixtures to stimulate the body.

The flavor and color of calendula account for its widespread use in cooking, particularly soups, cheeses and salads.

The volatile oils in calendula stimulate blood circulation and induce sweating, thus aiding fevers to break, and accelerate eruptions like measles or rashes. Calendula also increases urinating, aids digestion and acts as a general tonic. The herb's antiseptic value is likely related to its content of natural iodine.

CAT'S CLAW (Uncaria tomentosa)

We keep hearing about the medical potential of plants growing undiscovered in the Amazon jungles of South America. One that is showing great potential as an healing herb has been brought to this country. It is called cat's claw, or una de gato, its Spanish name.

Scientific studies on cat's claw are in progress, but Indians native to the Amazon rain forest have long relied on this herb to heal a range of ills. Although many, many claims have been made for the various healing powers of cat's claw, studies on it are limited.

The herb does, however, seem to hold promise for enhancing the immune system and as an anti-inflammatory, meaning it may well deliver relief from joint pain, like arthritis.

At this time, scientists have not isolated the active constituents of cat's claw in their quest to manufacture a patentable drug. In other words, the whole plant works very effectively, but there doesn't seem to. be one single ingredient that's responsible for its healing powers.

If you have arthritis, you may want to try cat's claw, particularly if other things you have tried for inflammatory conditions have proved unsuccessful.

One caution: natives of Peru reportedly use cat's claw for birth control, so please don't take it if you are attempting to become pregnant.

DONG QUAI (Angelica sinensis)

This fragrant perennial herb grows in China, Korea, and Japan. The root of the plant is described as having a head, body and tail to correspond with the herb's various applications.

The reputation of dong quai in Asia is second only to ginseng. Regarded as the ultimate, all-purpose woman's tonic herb, it is used for almost every gynecological complaint, from regulating the menstrual cycle and treating menopausal symptoms, such as hot flashes caused by hormonal changes, to assuring a healthy pregnancy and easy delivery. Chinese women have used dong quai for centuries to stop painful menstrual cramps caused by uterine contractions.

Herbalists today use dong quai for menopausal symptoms such as hot flashes, PMS, and to stimulate regular menstruation when women go off birth control pills.

Scientific investigation has shown that dong quai

produces a balancing effect on estrogen activity. The herb, rich in vitamins and minerals, has also been used to promote blood circulation and correct anemia in both sexes, as well as to treat insomnia, lower high blood pressure, and to alleviate constipation.

Most recently, studies involving dong quai have indicated that the herb regulates irregular heart beat, may help prevent heart disease, and acts as an immunostimulant to suppress tumors.

ECHINACEA (Echinacea angustifolia)

Resembling a black-eyed Susan, echinacea or purple coneflower is a North American herbaceous perennial that is also called snakeroot because it grows from a thick black root which Indians used to treat snake bites, indicative of the blood-cleansing quality attributed to this herb.

Native American tribes of the Plains States region are known to have used echinacea for medicinal purposes, notably as an antispasmodic or analgesic (pain killer). Indians also used the juice of the plant to bathe burns, the root to treat toothaches and sore throats, as well as for colds and flu. They would sprinkle the herb over a burning fire for "sweats" for purification purposes. During the 1920s, echinacea was one of this country's most popular plant drugs. Herbalists have long appreciated the healing benefits of echinacea as an effective antiviral and as a blood purifier to cure a host of ailments, including rheumatism, psoriasis, dyspepsia, gangrene, tumors, eczema and hemorrhoids.

Echinacea is regarded as a potent immunostimulator and as such has been used to treat such ailments as herpes, infections, candida and cancer. The herb has also been used to help restore normal immune function in cancer patients undergoing chemotherapy.

Studies have shown echinacea prevents the formation of an enzyme which destroys a natural barrier between healthy tissue and damaging organisms, such as herpes and influenza viruses. The herb is the most popular flu and cold remedy in Germany.

ELDERBERRY (Sambucus canadensis)

This herb has been intertwined with human history from the very beginning. Traces of elderberry have been found in Stone Age sites. It provided the wood for Christ's cross. Judas hung himself from an elder tree. Seventeenth century herbalist John Evelyn so highly regarded the elderberry, he called it a remedy "against all infirmities whatever." Gypsies agreed, calling it the "healingest tree on earth." Hippocrates wrote of its value as a purgative. One of Shakespeare's characters referred to it as "the stinking elder." There is even one growing outside of Westminster Abbey, planted there for its mystical ability to ward off evil spirits and disease.

Elder was widely used by several American Indian tribes. The Houmas boiled bark for use as a wash for inflammations. The Menominees used the dried flowers to brew a tea to reduce fevers. And the Meskivakis made tea from the root bark as an expectorant, and to treat headaches. Cooked elderberries were prepared as a drink by some tribes for neuralgia, sciatica and back pain, while others used the leaves in sweat baths to induce profuse sweating which brought relief from rheumatism pain. Scientific evidence exists that a substance in elderberries does in fact stimulate perspiration.

Externally, the herb has been used to relieve skin inflammation such as burns, rashes, and eczema. Elderberries are a good source of vitamins A, B, and C, plus flavonoids.

The berries are also the source of popular elderberry wine, regarded by many as a tonic, and the cooked berries are main ingredients for pies and jams. Most recently, new evidence was found to indicate remarkable value in an elderberry extract in the treatment of the flu virus.

EPHEDRA (Ephedra sinica)

This herb goes by the American names of cowboy tea and squaw tea, reflecting its use by early pioneers and Mormon settlers who used it primarily for asthma relief. It is also called Mormon tea, since it is brewed as a pleasant piney substitute for coffee and black tea, which Mormons avoid. The tea was made from powder derived from the dried green twigs of the shrub.

The Chinese name for ephedra is ma huang. The Chinese species of the herb grows in the Inner Mongolia region of China. Ephedra has been used in the Orient for nearly 5,000 years to treat asthma and upper respiratory symptoms such as coughs, as well as to reduce fevers and treat allergic skin reactions, such as hives.

Imported from China and cultivated in dry regions of North America, ephedra contains an alkaloid called ephedrine which provides effective decongestant, bronchodilator, antiasthmatic, and antiallergic functions. A synthetic version of ephedrine called pseudo-ephedrine is an ingredient found in many over-the-counter cold and allergy medications.

Ephedra has also been found to promote weight loss. This is due to its fat-metabolizing ability and to the fact that it suppresses appetite—an effect that is enhanced when it is combined with caffeine.

EUCALYPTUS (Eucalyptus globulus)

Native to Australia, where they account for 75 percent of the vegetation, eucalyptus trees are tall, graceful trees with slender, silvery leaves and creamy bark. Eucalyptus leaves are the dietary mainstay of koala bears, and humans use eucalyptus oil for a wide variety of medicinal purposes.

It is the aborigines of Australia who were first to discover that eucalyptus oil possesses medicinal properties. The most popular application of eucalyptus oil is for respiratory ailments. Used in a vaporizer, it doesn't take long for the volatile oils to help you breathe more freely and relieve the symptoms of a cold, chronic bronchitis, or asthma.

Eucalyptus oil (eucalyptol) is an effective expectorant used in many commercial drops or lozenges and in liquid preparations to loosen mucus from the nose and lungs and relieve upper respiratory discomfort. Distilled from leaves, the volatile oil is also used as a germicide.

Applied to the skin, eucalyptus oil increases the flow of blood to the area, bringing warming relief from stiffness and swelling, arthritis and rheumatism. The oil also possesses antiseptic qualities useful in the treatment of both respiratory infections and skin diseases. When aged, the oil forms ozone, a form of oxygen that will specifically destroy bacteria, fungi and certain viruses.

FEVERFEW (Chrysanthemum parthenium)

The name of this hardy biennial or perennial herb suggests its early use to bring down a fever. The ancient Greek herbalist, Dioscorides, used the herb to treat arthritis and also believed it helped regulate the uterus during the process of childbirth.

In the lengthy history of this herb, it has been used as an aromatic to ward off disease, for toothaches, as an insect repellent, and against a variety of ailments including kidney stones, constipation, arthritis, infant colic, and vertigo.

Perhaps the most effective modern-day application of feverfew is for headaches, but, as early as 1649, Culpeper noted that feverfew "is very effectual for all pains in the head." Later, in 1772, another famous herbalist, John Hell, wrote, "in the worst headache, this herb exceeds whatever else is known." But it wasn't until 1978 when British newspapers reported that a woman had cured her migraines with feverfew that medical researchers decided to examine the medicinal value of the herb. In 1980, *Lancet,* the highly respected British medical journal, reported that the herb shared properties with aspirin. Then in 1985, the *British Medical Journal* reported another study confirming that feverfew helps alleviate the pain of migraines. Three years later, *Lancet* confirmed the efficacy of feverfew in treating migraines. Once again, pharmaceutical companies have worked feverishly (no pun intended) to isolate the active ingredients of feverfew and turn it into a synthetic patent medicine—but with no success. It is the synergistic combination of ingredients in the feverfew plant that brings on such effective migraine relief.

Feverfew works to inhibit the release of two inflammatory substances—serotonin and prostaglandins—both believed to contribute to the onset of migraine attacks. It also appears that compounds in feverfew serve to make muscle cells less responsive to certain chemicals in the body that trigger migraine muscle spasms. Curiously, feverfew works only for migraines and not regular headaches.

GARLIC (Allium sativum)

Though it is best known as a culinary herb or vampire retardant, the medicinal benefits and claims for garlic are prodigious and worthy of the appellation "wonder drug among all herbs." Throughout recorded history, garlic has been used all over the world for a wide variety of conditions. In folk medicines it has been used for the plague, coughs, tuberculosis, diarrhea, as an antiseptic, to promote kidney function, as a blood cleanser, to kill intestinal parasites, and to prevent heart disease and cancer. It is also used as an antibiotic and antifungal.

Garlic is noted in ancient Chinese writings, mentioned in the Bible and in Homer's *Odyssey*, and has been found in the ancient tombs of Egypt. The Egyptians, incidentally, are said to have fed garlic to the slaves building the Pyramids to give them extra strength and nourishment.

Louis Pasteur discovered that garlic cloves would kill microorganisms in a petri dish. While working as a missionary in Africa, Dr. Albert Schweitzer used garlic to treat cholera, typhus, and amoebic dysentery. During both world wars, before the advent of antibiotics, garlic juice was daubed on infected wounds as a disinfectant to prevent gangrene. The Soviet Army relied so heavily on garlic that it earned the designation "Russian penicillin."

Modern-day research helps explain the broad applications of this "miracle" herb. The same component that gives garlic its strong odor is the one that destroys or inhibits various bacteria and fungi. This component is allicin, which, when garlic is crushed, combines with the enzyme allinase and results in antibacterial action equivalent to one percent penicillin. Garlic is reported to be even more effective than penicillin against typhus disease. It works well against both strep and staph bacteria, and the organisms responsible for cholera, dysentery and enteritis.

The irritating quality of garlic's volatile oil, readily absorbed into the bloodstream, may explain its use for respiratory problems by opening up lungs and bronchial tubes.

On top of everything else it does, this fascinating herb has been found to inhibit tumor cell formation and is under further investigation by the National Cancer Institute for its cancer-inhibiting qualities.

Please be aware that cooking garlic diminishes its potency, but several full-strength supplements and combinations of garlic are commercially available.

GINGER (Zingiber officinale).

It is the knotty branched root of this tropical perennial that is used for medicinal purposes as well as a pungent condiment. The Chinese have used ginger medicinally for well over 2,000 years. It is primarily employed to treat gastrointestinal disorders, particularly the removal of gas, colic, and indigestion. The herb possesses the ability to calm an upset stomach and to stop gripping and cramping in the abdominal and intestinal areas.

Ginger is a very effective and safe antinauseant, acting to prevent the symptoms of motion sickness and "morning sickness" in pregnant women including vomiting, dizziness and cold sweats. Drinking tea containing ginger for colds and asthma has long been a popular American remedy.

Ginger is a mild stimulant, promoting good circulation. Laboratory tests indicate ginger will lower cholesterol levels and inhibit the clotting and aggregation of blood.

A few drops of warmed ginger oil in the ear can soothe earaches. Grated ginger mixed with a little oil and applied to the scalp helps remedy dandruff. Ginger has also been credited with relieving headache and toothache pain.

GINKGO (Ginkgo biloba)

Ginkgo biloba is the Earth's oldest living tree species, traced back more than 200 million years. The tree itself can live 1,000 years, reaching over 100 feet high and 4 feet in diameter. The medicinal use of this "living fossil" goes back nearly 5,000 years.

An extract of ginkgo offers significant benefit to people with impaired blood flow to the brain. Symptoms of this cerebral insufficiency, commonly associated with aging, include short-term memory loss, headache, tinnitus (ringing in the ears), vertigo, and depression. Due to its high flavonoid content, ginkgo also improves circulation throughout the whole body, resulting in an increase in oxygen and blood sugar utilization to all internal organ systems and lower extremeties, thereby addressing problems related to poor circulation such as phlebitis. This positive vascular effect also serves to treat symptoms of underlying arterial insufficiency, providing protection against the development of Alzheimer's disease, strokes and hearing loss. It is a valuable medicine for diabetics, who suffer from impaired circulation to the extremities.

Free radical scavenging and antioxidant effects have been attributed to ginkgo and, hence slowing the process responsible for premature aging and cancer.

Hemorrhoids have been successfully treated by taking ginkgo extract. In one study, 86 percent of patients reported bleeding and pain stopped.

The effects of ginkgo as an antiallergenic and as an antiasthmatic agent have been scientifically demonstrated.

GINSENG (Panax ginseng)

This small perennial herb is without doubt the most famous medicinal plant of China. It was the Chinese who first noted that roots of ginseng resemble the human body and interpreted this as a sign of a medicine that could enhance the whole of human health. A portion that looked like a man would bring a higher price than an entire bale of nondescript roots. The word ginseng literally means "root of man" and the botanical name of one type, panax, is derived from "panacea."

Ginseng has been in use in China for 5,000 years as a tonic and rejuvenator. A Soviet scientist dubbed ginseng an "adaptogen," for its unique ability to normalize or bring into balance whatever is out of balance in the body. For example, if blood sugar levels are low, or if blood pressure is too high, an adaptogen will bring them back to normal levels. Ginseng acts on the pituitary, working to regulate blood sugar, supports the adrenal glands, and generally promotes physical and mental alertness, increasing energy and stamina. Diminishing fatigue is one reason athletes find particular benefit from the use of this herb.

Ginseng is believed to increase women's level of hormones, and is consequently recommended for some women for menopausal symptoms.

The herb stimulates weight and tissue growth and thereby enhances the body's resistance to disease. It particularly benefits the digestive process and the lungs and therefore treats lack of appetite, chronic diarrhea, shortness of breath or wheezing and insomnia.

Studies have shown that ginseng not only inhibits the production of cancer cells, but actually converts the abnormal cells into normal ones.

The hormone-like structure found in ginseng's saponins has a stimulatory action on sexual function in males and females, which may support the herb's reputation for enhancing sexual desire.

GOLDENSEAL (Hydrastis canadensis)

Widely used by a number of Native American tribes, goldenseal is a broad spectrum herb with a reputation for great medicinal virtuosity and, as a result, has been recommended for the treatment of many conditions and ailments.

An infusion of the roots is made into a wash for sore eyes and for skin diseases. Other uses of goldenseal include treatment for indigestion, loss of appetite and liver problems. It has been available as a commercial medicine in North America and throughout Europe for well over a hundred years.

Goldenseal is primarily used to treat congestion and soothe inflammatory conditions of the mucous membranes that line the respiratory, gastrointestinal, digestive, and genitourinary tracts. Goldenseal owes its medicinal value to its high content of the alkaloids hydrastine, hydrastinine and the more well-known gerberine. These alkaloids produce a strong astringent, antibiotic and immune-stimulating effect on mucous membranes.

Antibacterial components in goldenseal have proven effective in the treatment of diarrhea.

One experiment with goldenseal extract on laboratory animals brought about a drop in blood pressure.

Goldenseal can be used as an external application to arms and legs in the treatment of disorders of the lymphatic system and blood vessels. One folk remedy calls for rubbing goldenseal tea on the skin to treat eczema and ringworm.

A component of goldenseal was found to have anticonvulsive effects on the uterus. Goldenseal can also soothe irritated gums, help prevent gum disease and treat canker sores.

The herb is commonly used for female ailments such as vaginitis, and a douche of goldenseal can help relieve fungal infections such as Candida.

HAWTHORN (Crataegus oxyacantha)

The brilliant red berries of the hawthorn tree hang in dense clusters from thorny branches and remain on the tree until after the leaves drop in autumn.

Since the 17th century, hawthorn has had a history of use for its positive effects on the cardiovascular system. Traditionally, this herb was involved in the treatment of digestive problems, insomnia, and sore throat. Both Asian and North American cultures used hawthorn for weight loss. It also works as a diuretic, assisting the body in the elimination of excess salt and water.

Hawthorn benefits the heart in three ways: 1) flavonoids in hawthorn work to increase oxygen utilization by the heart, 2) it increases enzyme metabolism and acts as a mild dilator of heart muscle, and 3) it acts as a peripheral vasodilator (dilates blood vessels away from the heart), thereby lowering blood pressure and relieving the burden placed on the heart.

Specific cardiac symptoms for which hawthorn may be called for include recovery from a heart attack, cardiopulmonary disease, high blood pressure, and irregular heartbeat.

Hawthorn in combination with digitalis is given for cardiac problems such as palpitations, angina, and rapid heartbeat (tachycardia). One experiment indicated a mixture of hawthorn and the herb motherwort might prove an effective preventive or treatment for heart disease. Components in hawthorn have been shown to lower cholesterol as well as the size of plaque in arteries.

KAVA KAVA (Piper methysticum)

This herb, a member of the pepper family, grows as a bush in the South Pacific. The first European to discover it was Captain James Cook while he was sailing the South Seas. It was consumed during Polynesian religious rites for its ability to relax and soothe the mind.

Kava is also used for its medicinal effects as a sedative, muscle relaxant, diuretic, and as a remedy for nervousness and insomnia. The herb is also used as a pain reliever and can often be used instead of NSAIDs. (drugs such as aspirin, acetaminophen and ibuprofen).

Studies have shown kava to be as effective in treating anxiety and depression as the prescription antianxiety agents known as benzodiazepines (such as Valium), but without the adverse side effects. In fact, while the benzodiazepines tend to promote lethargy and mental impairment, kava has been shown to improve concentration, memory and reaction time for people suffering from anxiety.

LAVENDER (Lavandula officinalis)

Considered by some to be the quintessential English garden herb, and highly regarded for its classic fragrance in fancy soaps, sachets and potpourris, lavender also is important as a medicinal herb.

Traditionally, the flowers or oil from this old-fashioned herb were used to protect clothes and stored linens from hungry moths. It was also perhaps one of the first air fresheners, often found in early sickrooms. The name "lavender" is actually derived from the Latin verb "to wash," and both Greeks and Romans would scent their baths with the herb. Lavender was an ingredient of aromatic spirits of ammonia, the smelling salts that prevented or relieved fainting spells.

In China, the herb is used in a cure-all oil they call White Flower Oil. It is used as a medicine for hysteria, hoarseness, toothaches, colic, and skin conditions such as eczema and psoriasis. Oil distilled from the perfumy flowers of lavender has applications as a stimulant, a tonic, for headache relief and for relief of intestinal gas. It has also been used to quiet coughs and was once used as a disinfectant for wounds. Applied as a compress, warm lavender tea or oil provides relief for neuralgic pains, rheumatism, sprains, and sore joints.

LICORICE (Glycyrrhiza glabra)

We think of this plant as a candy flavoring (even though most licorice is actually flavored with anise oil); however, the root and constituents of this herb provide a tremendous number of valuable medicinal properties.

Two thousand years ago, the Chinese ranked licorice "superior," which meant it could be used over a long period of time with no toxic effects. They used licorice as a tonic to combat fevers and as a remedy for infection. It is the single most-used herb in Chinese medicine.

Ancient Greeks used licorice as a thirst quencher and to relieve swelling caused by water retention. The Blackfoot Indians used steeped wild licorice leaves in water as an earache remedy. Dutch physicians tested licorice as an aid for indigestion, which led to the use of the herb to treat peptic ulcers.

Other medicinal applications for licorice have included treatment of fever, menstrual and menopausal problems, influenza, arthritis, irritated urinary or bowel passages, and hypoglycemia. Additionally, it has been used as a diuretic, laxative and antispasmodic.

The most common medical use of licorice is for treating upper respiratory ailments including coughs, hoarseness, sore throat, and bronchitis. The rhizomes and roots in licorice have a high mucilage content which, when mixed with water or used in cough drops or syrup, is soothing to irritated mucous membranes and contributes to its use as an expectorant.

Another component of licorice, glycyrrhizin, stimulates the secretion of the adrenal cortex hormone aldosterone, and has a powerful cortisone-like effect. In fact, one study found glycyrrhizin was as effective a cough suppressant as codeine, and safer. In Europe, this unique compound is used extensively for its anti-inflammatory properties, especially for Addison's disease and ulcers. It has exhibited antiviral activity and as a result is used in Japan to treat chronic hepatitis B.

MILK THISTLE (Silybum marianus)

This herb is a stout annual or biennial plant, found in dry, rocky soils. One of the active principles of milk thistle is the flavonoid silymarin, which has been shown to have a direct effect on the cells of the liver, enhancing the overall function of this critical organ.

The known medicinal value of milk thistle is almost exclusively to support the liver. The liver detoxifies poisons that enter the bloodstream, such as alcohol, nicotine, heavy metals (e.g., lead and mercury) and environmental pollutants such as carbon monoxide and pesticides.

To underscore the importance of the liver, it is the source of the bile necessary for the breakdown of fats. It is also where vitamins A, D, E, and K are stored. No wonder the liver is referred to as the body's "chemical factory," and that the silymarin in milk thistle is so important.

In countless scientific studies, silymarin is reported to have shown positive effects in treating nearly every known form of liver disease, including cirrhosis, hepatitis, necroses, and chemical or drug and alcohol-induced liver ailments.

Silymarin's remarkable ability to prevent liver destruction and support liver function is believed to be due to its ability to inhibit the factors responsible for liver damage coupled with the fact it works to stimulate production of new liver cells to replace the old damaged ones. In addition, silymarin acts as an antioxidant, with far greater free radical damage control than even vitamin E in the liver.

Other studies have found that milk thistle offers some protection against the toxic side effects of the pain-relieving drug acetaminophen (Tylenol), a popular analgesic medication.

VITEX/CHASTEBERRY (Vitex agnus castus)

Chasteberry (also called vitex) was at one time recommended as a means for reducing excessive sexual desire, hence the significance of the "chaste" name for the plant. It is for this alleged effect that chasteberry was also used as a spice at monasteries during the Middle Ages where it was called "Monk's pepper."

Traditionally, chasteberry was very popular in Europe as a woman's remedy for regulating the reproductive system, treating PMS and unpleasant side effects associated with menopause, such as hot flashes.

Research has revealed the presence of a volatile oil in chasteberry which tends to balance the production of women's hormones. This oil is believed to contain a progesterone-like substance, which could explain the herb's therapeutic effect in relation to PMS symptoms such as anxiety, nervous tension, insomnia and mood changes, as well as problems associated with menopause such as hot flashes, vaginal dryness, dizziness and depression. Compounds in chasteberry also produce positive results when treating endometriosis, migraines, edema in the legs, cramps, and some allergies. Chasteberry has also been used to treat irregular menstruation, heavy bleeding and fibroid cysts.

Chasteberry extract can also improve skin conditions like acne by balancing sex hormones.

THE MINTS (Mentha)

We're talking here about more than the mint from the garden patch used to freshen a tall glass of lemonade or a mint julep.

All mints have cool, refreshing properties, and they have been used since antiquity all over the world in cooking and for their medicinal value. There are countless varieties and species of mints and all are generally stimulating and relieve indigestion, but three stand out in the herbal medicine cabinet: peppermint, spearmint, and pennyroyal.

Peppermint: The leaves of this perennial are a deeper, richer color than the bright, vivid green of spearmint. This species is also more stimulating to the circulation and is a stronger remedy for alleviating flatulence, heartburn and indigestion. Rather than cool off with a cold beverage in summer, the Chinese refresh themselves with a hot peppermint tea which leaves them feeling cooler because the infusion brings more blood to the skin causing perspiration, which then evaporates away the heat of the body. A stronger tea can be instrumental in breaking a fever. Peppermint is excellent for heartburn, stomach ache, nausea, and migraines.

Among other volatile oils, peppermint contains menthol and therefore has a minor antiseptic quality and is used as a gargle for sore throats and to cleanse wounds. Have a cup of mint tea after a heavy or rich dinner, because menthol also stimulates the flow of bile to the stomach, which promotes digestion and relieves upset stomach.

A simple tea makes a good headache remedy and can be useful to relieve tension and insomnia.

Spearmint: Much like peppermint, spearmint is an aromatic stimulant used for mild indigestion, to cure nausea, relieve stomach spasms and bowel pains, flatulence, motion sickness, and heartburn.

Spearmint tastes different from peppermint, and is also not as strong due to the fact that it contains no menthol. For this reason, spearmint can be substituted for the stronger mint when small children or very old people are being treated.

Pennyroyal: This herb, referred to as the "lung mint," was used to treat coughs and colds. It promotes perspiration to the point it helps break a fever. American Indians utilized pennyroyal to relieve menstrual cramps, and herbalists have recommended this mint to induce menstruation and treat premenstrual syndrome (PMS). Because of its ability to induce menstruation, pennyroyal should not be used by pregnant women. Pennyroyal oil makes an excellent insect repellent for pets.

SAW PALMETTO (Serenoa repens)

Saw palmetto is a small scrubby palm tree native to the U.S. Atlantic coast from South Carolina down through Florida. The tea from the berries of saw palmetto has long been used to treat urinary conditions and has been highly regarded as a remedy for enlarged prostate for centuries. Indeed, saw palmetto was tagged the "plant catheter" due to its therapeutic effect on the neck of the bladder and the prostate in men.

An extract of the saw palmetto will decrease urinary frequency, especially during night, due to inflammation of the bladder and enlargement of the prostate. Reduced urinary flow, dribbling, and impotence are symptomatic of an enlarged prostate or benign prostatic hyperplasia (BPH).

BPH is thought to be caused by a dysfunction of a type of the male hormone testosterone. Saw palmetto extract works to prevent testosterone from converting into dihydrotestosterone, the hormone thought to cause prostate cells to multiply excessively, leading to enlargement of the prostate. It is when the prostate grows abnormally that it pinches the urethra and interferes with urination. Early and effective treatment is important because when the urethra becomes completely blocked, urine can back up into the kidneys, causing severe abdominal pain which calls for immediate medical attention.

Others believe saw palmetto stimulates and increases bladder contractions, which facilitates easier and less painful urine flow.

Preliminary evidence exists to also suggest saw palmetto may also aid those suffering from thyroid deficiency. Moreover, this herb is a good expectorant for use in clearing chest congestion and is used to treat coughs due to colds as well as asthma and bronchitis.

ST. JOHN'S WORT (Hypericum perforatum)

Squeeze the petals of the flower from this shrubby perennial and a blood-colored resin will ooze out, which may explain why, according to legend, this plant sprang from the blood of Saint John the Baptist when he was beheaded.

For centuries in Europe, St. John's wort has been utilized as a mild tranquilizer and a treatment for depression and anxiety. While synthetic psychotropic drugs manufactured to treat these symptoms are associated with significant side effects (constipation, impaired urination, drowsiness), St. John's wort extract at recommended dosages shows no adverse side effects.

St. John's wort is also a muscle relaxant and is used to treat menstrual cramps. It is widely used for insomnia, and in Europe it is a popular remedy for gastrointestinal disorders.

Externally, it is an antiseptic and painkiller for burns and other irritations of the skin. Ointments containing St. John's wort are used to treat rheumatism and sciatica.

Most recently, evidence has surfaced that indicates components in St. John's wort may inhibit the growth of retroviruses in animals, including HIV, the AIDS virus.

TEA TREE OIL (Melaleuca alternifolia)

The tea tree is a small tree native to Australia, where it is acclaimed for its broad medical applications, particularly those affecting the skin. Although used in throat lozenges and in toothpastes, the oil distilled from tea tree leaves is most used externally.

In 1930, a surgeon in Sydney, Australia first noted the positive effect of tea tree oil for cleaning and healing surgical wounds. It has subsequently been determined that tea tree oil exhibits significant antiseptic and antifungal properties as well as stimulating skin rejuvenation.

The established value of tea tree oil as a disinfectant, coupled with the fact that it possesses good penetration properties and is nonirritating, makes it useful for a vast number of conditions including acne, diaper rash, heat rash, athlete's foot, canker sores, corns, insect bites, ringworm, lice, mouth ulcers, boils, sore throat, burns, psoriasis, root canal treatment, dandruff, respiratory congestion, gingivitis, herpes and yeast infections.

Tea tree oil is available in many products such as toothpastes, shampoos, soaps, throat lozenges, hair conditioners and skin lotions, and is packaged in forms such as salves, ointments, gels and liniments. Use as directed on the label.

UVA URSI (*Arctostaphylos uva ursi*)

The leaves of this perennial ground cover, known as bearberry, have an extended record as a folk remedy, particularly in relation to urinary tract problems. It is said that the Chinese introduced Marco Polo to this herb when he was traveling in China. European herbalists in the 13th century recognized the healing benefits of uva ursi.

Before the development of synthetic diuretic and urinary antiseptic drugs, uva ursi leaves were the main medicine available for these applications. The Chinese, European, and American natives all adopted uva ursi as an herb for healing the kidneys, using the leaves and fresh berries for treating kidney stones, bladder infections, and incontinence. Some tribes also mixed uva ursi leaves with other herbs and honey as a longevity elixir.

The strong urinary antiseptic, diuretic and astringent qualities of uva ursi are attributable to the active constituents hydroquinone and arbutin, which, interestingly, possess a more potent effect working together than either acting separately.

Analysis has shown that uva ursi contains a substance known to soothe and speed repair of irritated tissues. The herb has also exhibited antiviral, antibacterial and antifungal as well as antiplaque actions.

WHITE WILLOW BARK (*Salix alba*)

The white willow was introduced into the United States from Europe, and is now found gracing rivers and streams throughout the country. The bark is the part of the willow used medicinally and is easily removed in the spring when the sap begins to flow.

Willows have been tapped since antiquity for pain relief and reduction of fever. Ancient manuscripts of Egypt, Greece, and Assyria refer to willow bark, and even Hippocrates recommended willow to counter pain.

People have chewed the leaves or the inner bark of willows in this family of plants for thousands of years, and all contain salicylic acid. This compound was originally used by the Bayer Company in Germany in the late 1890s to synthesize acetylsalicylic acid, otherwise known as aspirin.

Natural salicylic acid is nearly as potent as aspirin. However, the compound salicin from willow does not cause gastric or intestinal upset of bleeding as aspirin can. This is because the natural product does not block prostaglandins in the stomach or intestines.

WITCH HAZEL (Hamamelis virginiana)

Witch hazel is a name derived from an old English word for "pliant," and the branches of this deciduous tree are in fact limber and were used as archery bows. Witch hazel is used principally as a skin liniment and astringent. Available in extract form, its anti-inflammatory action helps soothe minor scrapes, cuts and bruises. Applied externally to varicose veins or hemorrhoids, it helps relieve the pain and itching that accompany these conditions. A decoction of the bark is used as a dandruff wash, and the extract is useful for insect bites and sunburn.

PART III
Growing and Using the Healing Herbs

CHAPTER 6

Preparing and Taking Herbs

Just the slightest crush releases the wonderful aromas of plants like mint in our gardens and kitchens. This is one of the simplest ways to sample the powerful essence of herbs, one we use all the time in our kitchens. Freshly chopped mint with our potatoes or dandelion leaves in salad are examples of how it's often easy to take herbs as food. Frequently, though, it's more convenient or appropriate to use a herbal preparation. Then the trick is to capture the essence in usable forms. The range of herbal preparations is wide, including, for example, ointments for external application and capsules to be swallowed.

However an herb is prepared, its effect is achieved by interaction with our body chemistry. The aim is to ensure absorption and uptake by the bloodstream. Once circulating in the blood, an herb exerts its specific influence on the body. The key to traditional use and the work of skilled herbalists has always been the use of an herb's effects to support the body's own natural efforts to recover. This is unlike the tendency of many modern drugs designed to suppress the body's responses and produce short-term comfort.

This is not to say herbs can't bring immediate relief, as anyone who has soothed sunburn with aloe or calmed a toothache with oil of cloves will tell you. It is more that herbal treatments are gentler and aligned to the body's own processes. Treatment of illness with herbs may well require a little more time than a "knock-'em-dead" blast say, of antibiotics, but will be without the same risk of side effects and with much more likelihood of tackling the root cause.

Different conditions suit different methods of treatment based on selection of the best route for absorption of the herb. Absorption can take place through the digestive system, the skin, the lining of the mouth, ear and the nose, as with inhalation of hot vapors. Herbs are widely available now in a diversity of forms. Best results are obtained from organically grown fresh herbs. They should be preserved by proper drying and storage, so always check the source and avoid pills packed with fillers.

Many preparations can also be homemade, although the strongest form, essential oils, are best bought. Review the choices and enjoy tailoring your selection to your own particular needs. Remember— use herbs as directed, following the same precautions as with any medicine and always consult your physician if you are already being treated for a condition.

DROPS AND SPOONFULS

Some of the best internal herbal preparations are liquid and include syrups and tinctures. Tinctures are preservative mixtures of the herb in alcohol and water. Alcohol not only helps herbs last longer, it is also a good solvent for many of their active components. A standard ratio is 1:5 of the herb to the fluid. An example would be 7 ounces (200 grams) of herbs to 4½ cups (1 liter) of alcohol such as vodka, although cider vinegar can be used instead if preferred. For homemade tinctures, place the herbs in a dark, screw-top jar and cover them with the alcohol. The mixture should be shaken twice daily and stored, tightly covered, in a warm place. Use a muslin cloth to strain the residue, squeezing well, after two weeks. Tightly stoppered dark bottles help prevent evaporation and destruction of constituents by light.

Tinctures are usually taken with water and are a very concentrated way to take herbs. Some people like to add them to teas or even compresses. Mixing a tincture with a little beeswax, cocoa butter, or olive oil is also a useful way to make an ointment. And syrups? These are in fact tinctures added to sugar—a sweet way to make the herb go down!

A NICE CUP OF HERB

Drinking herbal teas can be one of the most pleasurable and effective ways of getting herbs into your system, although the taste of some leaves a lot to be desired! Teas are actually infusions. Boiling water helps extract and dissolve some of the medicinal compounds of an herb. This is a particularly useful way to prepare herbs desired for their potent aromatic oils, compounds which give teas their strong aromas. Tea bags or tea leaves are made from the dried herb and are generally equivalent to three parts of the fresh plant. When no particular dose is sought, a herbal tea can become more of a tonic, or included as part of a remedy, rather than one on its own.

Whereas infusions mainly use the soft, above-ground parts of plants, decoctions are another method of producing drinkable herbs. Decoctions are usually made with the woodier parts of plants like roots and bark. The chopped herb is brought to boil for 10 to 15 minutes, then strained immediately. More volatile components are lost, but decoctions capture the mineral salts and bitter principles, which can lead to some "interesting" tastes and powerful healing!

TAKE ONE AS DIRECTED

Some herbal preparations are in capsule form, as with many supplements and medicines. Gelatin containers are filled with finely powdered herbs, oils or extracted juice, usually in a hypoallergenic form. On reaching the gut, the shell is broken down, releasing the contents for absorption.

Herbs also come in traditional pill, tablet or lozenge form. Mucilage, gum, dry sugar or other binders and fillers are mixed with the powdered herb or with oil to make tablets or lozenges. Lozenges can be sucked, allowing them to be taken by a small degree into the bloodstream directly through the blood vessels of the mouth, but largely, again, through the walls of the intestine.

Homeopathic and some other preparations of herbs involve solutions mixed with sugar bases to create small pills. These are then placed under the tongue where they dissolve. This is known as sub-lingual absorption and is useful because it bypasses the liver. Always hungry to fuel its own processes, the liver is the blood's first major "stop" on its route from the stomach, and it is sometimes helpful to direct absorption elsewhere first.

APPLY WITH CARE, RUB GENTLY . . .

Many conditions are relieved by direct absorption of herbs through the skin. Sometimes part of the plant itself is used as with fresh aloe or mugwort, rubbed onto skin troubled by poison oak. Tinctures in fatty or oily bases make ointments, while more fluid liniments are herb extracts mixed with oils or alcohol.

Herbs can also be wrapped in material to make poultices which are laid on the skin. You can make compresses with wads of material soaked in herb decoctions or infusions. Topical applications like these are very useful for treating localized conditions like cuts, sprains and aches.

Expert massage can also involve specific herbal treatments with extracts of essential plant oils as in aromatherapy. The general benefits of a good all-over rub with a perfumed oil have been recognized for centuries. There's also nothing like relaxing in a bath of herbal salts as a way to feel the benefits of herbs working from the outside in.

GREAT HERB COMBOS

On the herbalist's menu are many formulas or combinations of medicinal plants established over history as stronger or broader in their effects than treatment with a single herb. Passionflower and valerian are good examples. Both reduce tension and anxiety, and a combination produces a double action, a natural sedative for short-term use.

Scientific investigation goes on to prove the synergistic value of combining herbs, balancing or increasing their individual chemical effects. For instance, sedative herbs are often supported by more stimulating ones like damiana to enable the body chemistry to even out rather than to swing one particular way. Licorice is used with the laxatives senna and cascara. The latter can cause intestinal pain, but licorice, itself a mild laxative, contains anti-inflammatory chemicals and lowers stomach acid levels, thus protecting against the harsher effects of the other two herbs.

Herbal formulas used in this way help to achieve harmony in the body and make very effective remedies.

CHAPTER 7

Your Herbal First Aid Kit for the Home

Herbal Preparation	Disorder	Treatment
Arnica ointment, Arnica tincture	Sprains and bruises, burns, scalds, stings, and impetigo	Rub ointment gently onto unbroken skin or apply a compress of tincture
Calendula tincture, Calendula ointment	Minor cuts	Bathe with tincture and/or apply ointment to cut.
Echinacea tincture	Insect bites	Apply tincture to bite and take one dropperful in water.
Echinacea and goldenseal mixture	Infections, flu and common cold	2-4 dropperfuls in water every 4 waking hours.
Herbal throat spray (with echinacea, goldenseal, and licorice, plus)	Sore throat	Spray back of throat as indicated on container.

Herbal Preparation	Disorder	Treatment
Ginger tea	Nausea	3-4 cups daily.
Peppermint tea	Headaches	3-4 cups daily.
Tea tree oil	Toothache, gum and fungal infections	Apply oil to affected area.
Valerian root tincture	Insomnia	Take drops with water as directed on container.
White willow capsules	Headaches	1 capsule as needed.

CHAPTER 8

Healing Herbs You Can Grow in Your Home or Garden

"The fresher the better" is certainly true of herbs. Gathering from the wild is still possible, but should only be done with an expert guide and with care not to exhaust an area of any one plant. Indoor and outdoor cultivation at your own home can be an enjoyable and inexpensive way to create your own supply of healing and culinary herbs. Starting with seeds gives you a choice of many varieties and is much cheaper than buying the plants themselves. Several herbs make natural partners, repelling insects for example, or promoting plant health, so be alert to opportunities for companion planting.

In tending herbs, you will be following a worldwide, centuries-old tradition. With your own flowerpots or a garden and rich organic soil, you can grow your own mini-pharmacy and reap the benefits of better health, not to mention more flavorful food! Try your hand with some of the herbs listed below and consult organic gardening books for tips on organic soil preparation, pest and disease control, plant layout and propagation.

HERB OR WEED?

Remember to check if a "weed" is itself a useful herb, like dandelion, that is worth cultivating where it will not smother other plants. However, plants such as bindweed, couch grass, creeping buttercup, ground elder and creeping thistle are all best removed as soon as they appear. They're also no good for composting.

HARVEST TIME

Many are the witch's brews that call for strange herbs picked at dawn or by the light of the moon. Actually, both seemingly strange practices make scientific sense because many of the medicinal compounds found in plants are volatile. This means they are evaporated by the sun's heat, so they are at their greatest concentration in plants before the sun is high in the sky. If you can, pick your herbs as soon as the dew has evaporated.

LEAVES AND FLOWERS

Pick leaves and flowers early in the morning, being careful not to bruise them. Flowers are usually best harvested as soon as possible after they have fully opened. For culinary purposes, leaves can be picked any time from a green and healthy plant. For medicinal purposes, however, leaves are usually best collected when flowers are in bud and before any have fully opened. Remember to shake off any insects.

GETTING TO THE ROOTS

Roots contain their greatest concentration of useful substances at the end of the growing season. Collect them at this time, discarding any that are damaged at all. Do not soak roots before drying, but wash them thoroughly to remove all soil.

DRYING HERBS

Always dry your harvest in the shade to avoid extreme temperatures. Try to disturb the plants as little as possible, although herbs dried on paper or trays will need to be turned occasionally. Small quantities can be dried on sheets of paper in a well-ventilated closet or on baking trays in a cool oven with the door open. For larger amounts, a warm, airy and shady space is needed. Herbs can be dried flat on large sheets of paper or on nets or stretched muslin. String up bunches of herbs well away from walls.

Dry small roots whole, but cut large ones into two or more pieces lengthwise. Thread root pieces on a string and hang them up to dry. Remove the outer coat of bulbs and slice before drying. When collecting bark, scrape off the outer layer, then peel away the inner layers, which can be dried in sunlight (except black cherry which needs shade). Temperatures should be *no higher* than 85-95° F for plants and leaves, 115° F for roots and 100° F for bulbs.

Leaves and stems are considered to be dry when they are brittle, breaking readily. Petals are ready when they rustle but do not crumble. Thick roots will chip with a small hammer, but most will snap. Three to seven days is a rough guide for most herbs, which will weigh about one-eighth of the fresh plant weight, but still smell and taste very much like it.

STORING HERBS

Herbs like tarragon, marjoram and thyme can be kept whole for bouquets garnis. Bay leaves, too, are good whole in soups and stews. Small flowers are also best kept intact, although marigold petals can be pulled off if preferred. With stalks removed, crush your dried herbs with a rolling pin or grinder or use a sieve for feathery herbs like dill.

Herbs deteriorate when exposed to oxygen and/or light. For this reason they must be stored in airtight, opaque containers. Dark glass jars with tight-fitting lids are best. For everyday use, keep small quantities in separate containers to lessen the exposure of your main stock to air and light. Don't forget to label each container, and dating them is a good idea, too. Keep herbs in a dark, cool closet or cupboard.

SOME FAVORITE HOME-GROWN HEALING HERBS

ALOE (Aloe spp.)

Type: Perennial. Many species. **Soil and situation:** Average, well-drained, full sun to light shade. **Spread/Height:** Up to several feet spread, up to 2 feet height, with very long stems. **Propagation:** From suckers or offshoots removed when 1-2 inches on indoor plant, 6-8 inches on outdoor plant. **Flower:** Yellow/orange-red, tubular, on stalks along a stem. **Leaves:** Pale, grayish-green, rubbery, long, spiky. **Harvest:** Older, outside leaves.

Aloe requires a minimum temperature of around 41°F and is frequently grown as a pot plant indoors, where it can thrive for years. When propagating, it's often best to dig up the plant, remove the suckers and then re-pot. Keeping a pot on the kitchen windowsill provides a simple remedy for minor burns and cuts and is always handy. Use scissors to cut off the end of a leaf, slice it down the middle and scrape out the clear gel. The gel is wonderfully soothing and is also used to help heal sunburn, itching and rashes. Aloe is a major constituent of many skin and hair preparations, but fresh aloe produces the best results. Josephine, wife to the emperor Napoleon, used a milk-and-aloe lotion to preserve her complexion. Indeed, aloe is said to help clear oily and acned skin. Some find aloe slightly drying, but mixing with a little vitamin E may prevent this.

CATNIP (Nepeta cataria)

Type: Perennial. **Soil and situation:** Average, well-drained, full sun to partial shade. Sow: Difficult with tiny seeds—see "propagation." **Height:** 1-3 feet **Propagation:** 4-inch stem sections rooted in moist medium. **Flower:** Small, tubular, white with purple-pink spots, massed in spikes, summer. **Leaves:** Oval, tooth-edged, gray-green with downy underside. **Harvest:** Tops and leaves when in full bloom.

Cats seem to get quite a high from the aroma of this plant, but don't go looking for the same effect on yourself—our brains are wired to respond differently to the chemicals in catnip! This mild herb, listed in the *U.S. Pharmacopoeia* from 1842 to 1882, has long been used to treat illness in children. Brewed as a hot infusion, catnip promotes sweating and is good for infectious diseases such as measles as well as colds and flu. Soothing to the nervous system, it helps restless children get to sleep. This may be because the chemical structure of a major part of catnip's volatile oil is related to valepotriates, the known sedatives found in valerian. Catnip also has a calming effect on the stomach, and is helpful for colic, flatulence and diarrhea. Its sharp flavor made catnip an ingredient in Roman salads, and catnip tea was very popular in England before foreign varieties cornered the market.

EVENING PRIMROSE (Oenothera biennis)

Type: Biennial. Many other species. **Soil and situation:** Stony, dry, full sun. **Sow:** Late summer. **Spread/**

Height: 2 x 5 feet. **Flower:** Mid-late summer, on spikes, large, bright yellow. **Leaves:** Shiny, long, pointed. **Harvest:** Flowers, seeds, root.

Studies have given substantial support to the use of evening primrose in treating a number of disorders, from dry eyes and brittle nails to hyperactivity in children, premenstrual syndrome, alcoholic poisoning, acne, overweight, rheumatoid arthritis, and coronary artery disease. Evening primrose is very high in essential fatty acids, especially one called GLA which is needed for the production of a hormone-like substance, PGE1, which has a range of beneficial effects in the body. The whole plant is edible. Try a tincture, or infusions can be made with 1 teaspoon of the plant to one cup of water to be taken, one mouthful at a time, once a day. Exercise caution, though, as evening primrose is not recommended for epileptics, and some people have reported sensitivities to the plant.

FENNEL (Foeniculum vulgare)

Type: Semi-hardy perennial. **Soil and situation:** Very well-drained, full sun. **Sow:** Mid-summer, fall. **Spread/ Height:** 3 × 4-6 feet. **Flower:** Small, yellow, on umbrella of stalks, midsummer. **Leaves:** Deep green, thin, feathery, aromatic. **Harvest:** Ripe seeds, young leaves, green stems.

Take care of fennel, for it is vulnerable to harm from certain plants including wormwood, which can inhibit seed germination and stunt its growth, while coriander will prevent seeds from forming. You should also make this herb a loner in your garden because it can damage other plants like bush beans, caraway, tomatoes and kohlrabi. Fennel, with its refreshing anise-like flavor, has long been known as a digestive aid included in recipes by the Greeks, Romans and Anglo-Saxons before spreading even further abroad.

Add fennel to soups and salads. Drink fennel tea for indigestion and heartburn and serve it to babies to relieve their colic. It's also an ancient remedy used to promote the flow of milk in nursing mothers. Fennel eyewash is recommended for tired, sore eyes and the oil is antispasmodic and antibacterial, although not recommended for those with allergies or skin sensitivities.

GARLIC (*Allium sativum*)

Type: Perennial bulb. Many varieties. **Soil and situation:** Well drained, rich to medium, full sun to partial shade. **Height:** 1 foot. **Propagation:** Split into cloves. Plant early spring or fall. **Flower:** Very small, white to pinkish, late summer. **Leaves:** Long, flat, pointed. **Harvest:** Leaves, early summer; bulbs, late summer.

Many gardeners believe roses benefit from garlic planted close by and, of course, they're a good idea if you're having trouble with vampires! In reality garlic wards off many diseases. Research shows that eating garlic protects against heart disease by lowering cholesterol and other fats, and by reducing blood-clotting activity and hypertension. Garlic is also good for intestinal infections. Take grated garlic mixed with honey for coughs. Apply garlic to wounds to prevent infections. Of course, you can also enjoy garlic's unique flavor in foods.

GERMAN CHAMOMILE (*Matricaria chamomilla*)

Type: Annual. **Soil and situation:** Most types, especially light. **Sow:** Late summer/fall. **Spread/Height:** 4 inches x 2 feet. **Flower:** From early summer, small, daisy-like. **Leaves:** Feathery, bright green. **Harvest:** Flowers when fully open.

This plant is known as the "doctor's physician" and is described by Germans as "capable of anything." An aid to plants, too, German chamomile repels flying insects and even helps improve onion crop yield. Chamomile flowers contain a lovely blue volatile oil called azulene, and its many effective compounds include two powerful antiseptics. Use externally for hair care, especially fair hair, in combination with soapwort. You can also steep 3-4 ounces in boiling hot water for 1 hour to make a relaxing bath mixture. Make a tincture for washes or compresses to soothe and aid the healing of rashes, burns and wounds.

Brew an infusion and drink chamomile as tea. This will aid nervous conditions, insomnia and neuralgia. Chamomile has also been shown to calm restless children. In fact, chamomile was the tea served to Peter Rabbit by his mother to soothe his aching stomach! It's a famous remedy for digestive upsets, including diarrhea and flatulence, with research proving it is anti-inflammatory, and antispasmodic. Chamomile is also used to prevent and treat ulcers.

GINGER (*Zingiber officinale*)

Type: Tropical biennial. **Soil and situation:** Container, indoors. Loam, sand, peat moss and compost in equal parts. Light shade, warmth, moisture and humidity. **Height:** 2-4 feet. **Propagation:** From rhizome. **Flower:** Rarely in cultivation. Dense spikes, yellow-green, purple spotted and striped. **Leaves:** Grass-like, long, pointed. **Harvest:** Root, 8-12 months after planting.

Ginger is a commercial crop throughout the tropics, supplying an international trade in culinary spices and herbal medicines that goes back thousands of years. For your own harvest, pull the mature plant from its pot, cut off the leafstalks and thinner, fibrous roots. Cut off as much of the main root as you can store and use. The remainder can be re-planted. Wrap your ginger first in a paper towel, then tightly in plastic wrap. Refrigerated, ginger will last for several months. Chew on a fresh stick to relieve a sore throat. Dry some, too, for dry ginger has slightly different chemical actions, traditionally making it more suitable for respiratory and digestive disorders.

All ginger is warming, but fresh ginger induces sweating and is said to be better for treating colds.

Studies have shown ginger provides much relief from nausea in early pregnancy at just 250 milligrams four times daily, and also from the pain, swelling and stiffness of both osteo- and rheumatoid arthritis, using doses from 500 to 4,000 mg daily. Cook Indian style and you'll soon exceed these doses! Daily amounts of 8 to 10 grams are regularly consumed in India where this herb continues to be very popular in both main dishes like curry and desserts such as crystallized ginger.

LAVENDER (Lavandula officinalis)

Type: Perennial shrub, evergreen. **Soil and situation:** Light, well-drained, calcareous, full sun. **Sow:** Early spring or fall without heat. **Spread/Height:** 2 x 2 feet 8 inches. **Propagation:** Spring—softwood cuttings, fall—hardwood cuttings. **Flower:** Mid-summer, mauve. **Leaves:** Narrow, gray-green. **Harvest:** Flowers, mid/late summer.

Use lavender for hedging and cut it back when it has finished flowering. Lavender takes its name from the Latin verb "to wash" and was used by Romans and Greeks to create relaxing, scented baths. Widely known for its lovely scent, lavender is also used in steam inhalation against coughs, colds and chest infections. Make an infusion of lavender for the same conditions as well as for tension, anxiety, stomach and headaches. The oil is antibacterial, helpful for healing cuts, and is one of the best remedies for stings and burns. A few drops used in massage help to relax muscles and ease pain. As with all plant oils, do not take lavender oil internally.

LEMON BALM (Melissa officinalis)

Type: Perennial, evergreen. **Soil and situation:** Average, well-drained, sun or semi-shade. **Sow:** Late spring. **Spread/Height:** 2 feet x 2 feet 8 inches. **Propagation:** In spring, layering, root division, cuttings. **Flower:** Small, white to pink or yellowish, in clusters, summer. **Leaves:** Broad, oval, toothedged, lemon fragrance. **Harvest:** Leaves and stems in growing season.

Lemon balm is a good bee plant, its official name coming from the Greek word for "bees." Strangely, it is also considered to be a good insect repellent, used to keep flies off food and away from fires.

Harvest this herb by cutting off the entire plant two inches above the ground. It needs to be dried within two days of harvesting for it can quickly turn black. A tip from Shakespeare's *Merry Wives of Windsor* is to rub lemon balm into wood, letting its fragrant oils act as a natural equivalent to lemon-scented furniture polish. You can also make a pleasant tea with this herb as a remedy for colds, flu, depression, headache and indigestion. In fact, lemon balm has been recommended for centuries because "it makes the heart merry."

Analysis shows the effects of the plant's volatile oils are due to antispasmodic and strong sedative properties which also make lemon balm helpful for promoting menstrual periods and relieving menstrual cramping. Its polyphenols may be responsible for its antiviral effects, demonstrated against mumps and other viruses. Relax in a cleansing, steamy bath mixture of lemon balm and use it as an acne rinse. Chop it up for culinary use, too, with salads, chicken and lamb. Drink the liqueurs, Benedictine and Chartreuse and you'll be downing lemon balm, too!

MEADOWSWEET (Filipendula ulmaria)

Type: Perennial. **Soil and situation:** Moist, rich, sun or semi-shade. **Sow:** Spring or fall. **Spread/Height:** 1 x 2-3 feet. **Propagation:** Divide roots in spring. **Flower:** Summer, cream, clustered. **Leaves:** Dark green. **Harvest:** Flower heads, leaves, roots in the fall.

Meadowsweet is a good plant to grow by water. Its active compounds include substances like those found in aspirin, antioxidants, vitamin C and sugar. Science shows us how meadowsweet's particular chemical package made it a safe remedy for hundreds of years for conditions like children's diarrhea, rheumatism and fevers. Its anti-inflammatory constituents on their own could cause gastric bleeding, yet it also contains tannin and mucilage which seem to act as buffers, preventing the adverse effect. Meadowsweet also acts as an antiseptic diuretic, aiding the excretion of uric acid. Make a hot infusion to induce sweating, an old-fashioned but useful treatment for fevers. Boil two tablespoons of the plant or dried rootstock in one cup of water and take one cup a day as a remedy. You can also use this decoction as a wash for wounds or sore eyes.

PARSLEY (Petroselinum crispum)

Type: Biennial. **Soil and situation:** Rich, moist, well-drained, sun to semi-shade. **Sow:** Spring inside, warm. Mid-summer outside, full sun with shelter. **Spread/Height:** 1 foot 4 inches x 2 feet. **Propagation:** Allow to self-seed. **Flower:** Tiny, greenish yellow in umbrella clusters, summer. **Leaves:** Dark green, feathery. **Harvest:** Leaves, seeds, root.

You may know that parsley is a useful breath sweetener, but you probably haven't heard how it used to be sprinkled on corpses as a deodorizer! Its high chlorophyll content helps it eat up internal odors (including garlic), and its oils are naturally aromatic, leading to its popular use in bouquets garnis and as a garnish. Parsley is said to be good in a vegetable patch because it is supposed to repel some insects.

An excellent source of vitamin C, usefully packaged with iron, a nibble of parsley makes sense when you're under the weather. You'll also be taking in several B vitamins, vitamin A, calcium, manganese and phosphorus. Its role as a nutritional mini-powerhouse backs up its medicinal effects as a diuretic suitable for treating urinary infections and fluid retention. Because it helps expel uric acid, parsley is a remedy for gout and the root has laxative properties.

Pregnant women should avoid large amounts of parsley. On the other hand, the chemistry of parsley strengthens uterine muscles and increases breast milk. Parsley is a digestive aid and as a tincture, two to 15 drops in water, as needed, it makes a treatment for nausea. Cosmetically, parsley infusions are soothing and cleansing and can be used as a hair rinse. Parsley oil is found in many cosmetics, shampoos, soaps and skin lotions. If you can, freeze your parsley as this is said to give better results than simply drying.

ROSEMARY (Rosmarinus officinalis)

Type: Perennial shrub. Many decorative subspecies. **Soil and situation:** Calcareous, well drained, full sun, sheltered from wind. **Sow:** 75-80°F in seed tray. **Height:** 5 feet 8 inches. **Propagation:** From early summer, cuttings of non-flowering shoots. **Flower:** Late spring, pale to deep blue. **Leaves:** Leathery, thin, gray-green, oily, aromatic. **Harvest:** Leaves as needed.

Rosemary's traditional companion is sage. Plant it with carrot, too, as it repels carrot fly. It is an excellent hair tonic, and its refreshing scent leads to its use in cosmetics and perfumes. Ancient Greeks even made rosemary garlands to strengthen their memories at exam times! Medicinally, rosemary has many uses and is listed officially in the *U.S. Pharmacopoeia.* Even as recently as World War II, French hospitals burned juniper berries with rosemary leaves to kill germs. The oil, which, like many essential oils, is antifungal and antibacterial, is part of several liniments for rheumatism and can be applied directly to the head to relieve headaches. Enjoy rosemary with, say, a dish of lamb, and you will be reducing flatulence, stimulating your digestion, liver, gall bladder and circulation. Infusions of rosemary, of course, are used for the same reasons, as well as for treating painful menstruation. Use caution with rosemary, for the undiluted oil should not be taken internally.

SAGE (Salvia officinalis)

Type: Perennial shrub. **Soil and situation:** Well-drained, calcareous, full sun. **Sow:** Late spring. **Spread/Height:** 1 foot 8 inches × 1-2 feet. **Propagation:** Cuttings, spring. **Flower:** Tubular, purple, pink, blue or white, early summer. **Leaves:** Gray-green, velvety, aromatic. **Harvest:** Leaves.

Sage is a beneficial companion plant in general and especially for rosemary and vines. In addition, it repels cabbage moths and a number of other harmful flying insects. American Indians used the fragrant, silver-green sagebrush of the American chaparral as a toothbrush, cleanser and remedy with bear grease for skin sores, but its bitter taste rules it out of competition with the cultivated Mediterranean variety for culinary use.

Named from the Latin "to save," sage has been associated for centuries with longevity. The Chinese would even trade up to four times their fine green tea for European sage. As you stuff that turkey, you're dispensing a long-esteemed remedy for sore throats, colds, indigestion, hot flashes and painful periods. Mix sage tea with a little cider vinegar for relief from throat disorders like tonsillitis. Use the tea as a mouthwash for infected gums and mouth ulcers. Feel its volatile oil work as it boosts digestion. It will also stop sweating and is reputed to dry up the flow of breast milk. Sage is also used for treating amenorrhea and painful periods.

This wide range of applications has its origins in the variety of substances found in sage. Besides its powerful oils, sage contains estrogenic compounds, antibacterial agents, antioxidants and tannins. Do note, though, that sage should only be taken as remedy for a week or two at a time, since it has another substance, thujone, which can have potentially toxic effects. But when you turn to sage in the kitchen, remember its extensive medicinal powers as you use it in dishes from soups and salads to meats, cheese and bread.

SWEET BASIL (ocimum basilicum)

Type: Tender annual. One of many varieties. **Soil and situation:** Fertile loam, sun. **Sow:** Spring inside, warm. Midsummer outside, full sun with shelter. **Spread/ Height:** 1 × 1-2 feet. **Propagation:** Cuttings. **Flower:** Mid to late summer, white/purplish. **Leaves:** Delicate, clear green, aromatic. **Harvest:** Leaves as needed, stems before flowering.

The chopped leaves of basil are famous for their distinctive flavor in dishes like pesto. Its other main use is as an insect repellent! In Europe, it is grown in pots outside doors to deter flies. Plant it near tomatoes for the same reason. Basil is also recommended for gastric disorders such as stomach cramps and constipation. Steep 1 teaspoon of dried herb in ½ cup of water. Take 1-1½ cups a day, one mouthful at a time. You can even do as some residents of New Mexico and carry basil in your pockets to attract money!

CHAPTER 9

Aromatherapy Herbs

Has a whiff of something ever sent you back to childhood, a special occasion or the company of someone special? Such is the power of smell, harnessed even as a marketing tool, supermarkets creating the illusion of fresh bakeries and real estate agents filling vases, heating vanilla in the oven and brewing coffee! In plants, the source of their potent scents is essential oils. Such oils serve them as insect repellents or attractants, antibacterial and antifungal agents and often lends them a particular character. In perfumes, ointments and sprays they do the same for us! Essential oils act as stimulants or relaxants to humans, frequently providing a link from the physical to the emotional as the olfactory organs connect to the parts of the brain associated with emotions. Formal research is scant, but work done at Milan University gives scientific support to the observation that plant oils can lift our spirits, relieving anxiety and depression.

BREATHE DEEPLY AND RELAX

As volatile substances, plant oils are extracted by distillation or soaking. The result is highly concentrated products which are absorbed through the skin or, diluted, through inhalation. Direct, external use of essential oils dates back thousands of years to ancient Egypt and Greece, and the Far East. Hippocrates encouraged the burning of aromatic plants to prevent the spread of plague in ancient Athens. Gattefossé, an early French aromatherapist, recounted how, on impulse, he thrust his burnt hand into a bowl of lavender essence and found it healed extremely rapidly.

Today, we can choose an incense to burn, buy commercial vaporizers and visit steam baths. Do-it-yourself inhalation methods include mixing one or two drops of essential oil in a bowl of steaming hot water, then placing a towel over your head and around the bowl to catch the steam. Soak in a bath, too, where five or six drops have been dissolved in warm water.

Five or six drops of oil are appropriate for massage, the oils being diluted in two to five teaspoons of carrier oil such as almond, grape seed or soy. Massage with essential oils stimulates blood circulation, boosting their absorption. It also activates nerve endings, which aromatherapists believe then channel a reaction along nerves to the pituitary gland. The pituitary gland regulates the function of other glands, including the adrenals, and in this way influences whether we feel stressed or relaxed. This ties in with scientific analysis of several oils showing them to contain substances known to be stimulative or sedative in their effects.

Different oils are also reputed to produce different emotional effects, basil bringing cheer, catnip and rue inducing calm, and ylang ylang promoting sex and love, for example. Seek out *natural* essential oils. Keep in mind that natural oils are very highly concentrated and pack the power of the plant in a way synthetics cannot match. Choose your oil to suit, then pamper yourself with aromatherapy, one of the oldest health promotion measures known.

CHAPTER 10

Herbs for the Bath

For a wonderful addition to any bath, simply add a few drops of oil or a pint or so of a very strong infusion, strained, of your chosen herb to the bath water. One of the best and simplest herbal bath remedies is eucalyptus. Just on its own, this antiseptic herb brings relief from aches and pain, clears the head and sinuses and warms the body as it increases blood flow. You can also make an herb sachet to soak in the bath and smooth over your skin. Mix two cups of dried flowers, such as lime or chamomile, with one cup of fine oatmeal. Place them in the center of a piece of muslin about 16 inches square. Gather up the edges of the muslin, tying it up tightly with thread or string. Enjoy at least a ten-minute soak with herbal mixtures like those below.

SKIN SAVERS

To soothe dry, itchy or inflamed skin, try a bath mixture with a cold-pressed vegetable oil base. As well as relieving symptoms and helping to protect your skin, such oils provide a natural barrier to moisture loss. Avoid using corn or cottonseed oils as these are derived from crops usually heavily sprayed with pesticides and fungicides. Also avoid mineral oils, as they clog pores. Mix ½ cup of each of almond, safflower, soy, and sesame oils. Shake all these together with a drop or two of an essential oil such as tea tree which is a powerful skin disinfectant that penetrates and helps heal infected areas very well. Add two tablespoons to your bath using the full flow of the hot tap and take a luxurious soak.

Birch bark, chamomile, clovers, comfrey root, marshmallow root, pansy, seaweed, white willow, and wintergreen, are all recommended as calming herbs. For psoriasis, take a bath with comfrey root mixed with white willow bark.

SOAK AND REJUVENATE!

For an antistress bath, try a combination of comfrey leaf, linden, patchouli, sandalwood, and savory in equal parts. Comfrey works against signs of aging, due to its high allantoin content. Allantoin promotes the growth of bone and cartilage and connective tissue, the latter being essential to healthy skin. Sandalwood improves skin tone, and savory is stimulating. This is balanced by linden, a natural antiseptic and relaxant, helping to produce a fortifying, antistress, and fragrant bath.

An herbal mixture recommended especially for long-term, repeated use to keep skin young-looking and firm uses 1 ounce each of aloe, comfrey root, lavender, lemon thyme, peppermint, rosemary, and fresh or dried roses. A little of this assortment works well on the body in various ways. The proven benefits of comfrey are supplemented by the cooling, healing astringency of aloe and roses. Lavender has a calming, antibacterial action, working well against acne and puffiness, and is reinforced by the roses, which also hydrate the skin. The menthol in peppermint is cooling and anesthetic as well as stimulating to the blood flow in skin. Thyme eases aches and pains and acts as a mild deodorant. Emerge from a soak in these herbs feeling fresh, clean and alive!

CHAPTER 11

Make Your Own Potpourri

Forget the disinfectants and air fresheners in a can!
Go for natural, environmentally friendly fragrances instead. Simply hang up bunches of herbs chosen for
their scent and their effects on mood. Try your hand,
too, at combining dried herbs in potpourris, following
recipes like the one below, or make up your own. Tip
a little of each herb into a covered bowl to be exposed
when occasional scent is desired, or into an open container for continuous fragrance. Stir the herbs and
other ingredients together and sprinkle them with a
few drops of an oil with a complementary odor.

Bring the scents of a flower garden indoors with
five tablespoons of lavender flowers, three tablespoons
each of carnations and scented rose petals, one and a
half tablespoons each of chamomile flowers, helio-
trope flowers, salt, and orris root powder. A little rose
oil is a nice addition.

CHAPTER 12

Herbal Insect Repellents

The single most important reason that plants contain aromatic volatile oils is to repel insects! We can take advantage of this by using aromatic oils to repel pests, instead of the toxic petrochemical pesticides sold commercially. In fact, many of these substances can now be found at better plant and garden stores.

Pyrethrums, which come from plants in the chrysanthemum family, make potent insecticides as powder from the dried plants or spray infusions. Pyrethrum works by paralyzing insects and is so strong that prolonged contact can cause skin problems, so use it with care.

You can also make an infusion of 1 pound of elder leaves to 2 gallons of water as an effective aphid spray. And try a decoction of walnut leaves, six handfuls boiled for 20-30 minutes in one pint of water, to repel ants. Indoors, use southernwood, also known as garderobe (cothesguard), between sheets of tissue lain among clothes to keep moths away. Hanging bunches of herbs such as pennyroyal, rosemary, rue and tansy adds lovely scents to the summer air as they keep insects out of the house on summer evenings.

Venture out to flea-ridden grasses and the muggiest swamps wearing some of nature's own bug repellents! A short-term mosquito repellent is fresh elder. Simply rub the leaves on exposed parts, but be prepared to do this every twenty minutes. You can also make strong infusions of elder or chamomile to dab on frequently.

Citronella oil, made from the stone root plant, is a well known and longer-lasting bug deterrent. It also has a pleasant fragrance, and is much more effective and easier to apply than most store-bought insect repellents. Lavender oil is reputed to be similarly useful and has its own well-loved scent. Armed against bugs and perfumed as well—yet another typically effective, gentle and enjoyable result of using herbs!

Any of the plants with aromatic essential oils but especially pennyroyal, can also used as insect repellents.

CHAPTER 13

An Abbreviated Guide to Herbs and Illnesses

For	Use
Allergies	Ephedra, garlic
Arthritis	Cat's claw, arnica, feverfew, licorice, evening primrose, ginger
Cholesterol lowering	Garlic, ginger, hawthorn
Circulation	Ginkgo biloba, garlic, angelica, bilberry, calendula, ginger
Colds and flus	Echinacea, ephedra, garlic, goldenseal, elderberry
Cough	Licorice, ephedra, garlic, lavender
Depression, anxiety	Kava kava, St. John's wort
Digestion	Ginger, chamomile, the mints, fennel, angelica, licorice
Headache	Feverfew (migraine only), white willow bark, ginger, ginkgo, lavender, the mints
Heartburn	Licorice, the mints, fennel
Heart Strengthener	Hawthorn berries, garlic, dong quai

For	Use
Insomnia	Valerian, St. John's wort
Immune System Support	Echinacea, garlic, ginseng, angelica, cat's claw, goldenseal
Liver Support	Milk thistle
Lungs	Licorice, eucalyptus, garlic, ginseng, pennyroyal
Memory	Ginkgo biloba, kava
Menopause	Dong quai, vitex/chasteberry, angelica, licorice, ginseng
Pain	White willow bark, feverfew, arnica, licorice, aloe, calendula, cat's claw, echinacea, elderberry, kava, lavender
PMS	Vitex, dong quai, pennyroyal
Prostate	Saw palmetto
Sores, wounds, cuts and bruises, stings, bites and itches	Witch hazel, aloe vera, arnica, calendula
Urinary Tract	Uva ursi, saw palmetto
Vision	Bilberry

Sources and Resources

SOURCES

Barrie, N.D., "Effects of Garlic Oil on Platelet Aggregation, Serum Lipids and Blood Pressure in Humans," *Journal of Orthomolecular Medicine,* 1987, 2(1):15-21

Byrnes, P., "Wild Medicine," in *Wilderness,* The Wilderness Society, 1995, Vol.59, 210:28-33.

Farnsworth, N., et al., "Medicinal Plants in Therapy," *Bull World Health* Org., 1985, 63:965-981.

Fogarty, M., "Garlic's Potential Role in Reducing Heart Disease," *British Journal of Clinical Practice,* 1993, 47(2):64-65.

Hobbs, C., *The Echinacea Handbook,* Eclectic Medical Publications, Portland, OR, 1989.

Kowalchik, C., et al., *Rodale's Illustrated Encyclopedia of Herbs,* Rodale Press, Emmaus, Pennsylvania, 1987.

Lemley, B., Interview with Andrew Weil, *New Age Journal,* Dec. 1995:68.

Lust, J., *The Herb Book,* Bantam Books, New York, 1974.

Mabey, R., *The New Age Herbalist,* Collier Books, Macmillan Publishing Co., New York, 1988.

Macolo, N., et al., "Ethnopharmalogic Investigation of Ginger (Zingiber Officinale)," *J. Ethnopharmacol,* 1989, 27:129-140.

Mann, C., et al, "The Chemistry, Pharmacology, and Commercial Formulations of Chamomile," *Herbs Spices Med Plants,* 1985, 1:235-280.

Mindell, E., *Earl Mindell's Herb Bible,* Simon & Schuster/Fireside, New York, 1992.

Moore, Michael, *Medicinal Plants of the Mountain West,* Museum of New Mexico Press, Santa Fe, New Mexico, 1979.

Moore, Michael, *Medicinal Plants of the Pacific West,* Red Crane Books, Santa Fe, New Mexico, 1993.

Mowrey, Daniel B., Ph.D., *The Scientific Validation of Herbal Medicine,* Keats Publishing, New Canaan, CT, 1986.

Murray, M, *The Healing Power of Herbs,* Prima Publishing, California, 1995.

Rose, Jeanne, *Jeanne Rose's Herbal Body Book,* Perigree, Putnam Publishing, New York, 1976.

Tierra, Lesley, L.Ac., Herbalist, *The Herbs of Life: Health and Healing Using Western and Chinese Techniques,* The Crossing Press, Freedom, CA, 1992.

Vanderhoek, J., et al., "Inhibition of Fatty Acid Lipoxygenases by Onion and Garlic Oils. Evidence for the Mechanism by Which These Oils Inhibit Platelet Aggregation," *Bioch. Pharmacol.,* 1980, 29, 3:169-173.

Weiner, M., *Earth Medicine—Earth Food,* Fawcett Columbine, New York, 1980.

Werbach, Melvyn R. M.D., and Murray, Michael T, N.D., *Botanical Influences on Illness,* Third Line Press, Tarzana, California, 1994.

Willard, Terry, Ph.D., *The Wild Rose Scientific Herbal,* Wild Rose College of Natural Healing, Calgary, Alberta, 1991.

RESOURCES

For more information on herbal medicines contact the following organizations:
The American Botanical Council
P.O. Box 201660
Austin, TX 78720
(512) 331-8868

The Herb Research Foundation
1007 Pearl Street, Ste. 200
Boulder, CO 80302
(303) 449-2265

An excellent guide to alternative medicine health care professionals is *The Alternative Medicine Yellow Pages*, $12.95. It is also available in many bookstores. It is published by:

Future Medicine Publishing
98 Main Street, Ste. 209
Tiburon, CA 94920

For referrals to naturopathic physicians write or call:
American Association of Naturopathic Physicians
P.O. Box 20386
Seattle, WA 98102
(206) 323-7610

For referrals to Chinese Medicine Doctors, contact:
American Association of Acupuncture and
Oriental Medicine
4101 Lake Boone Trail, Ste. 201
Raleigh, NC 27607
(919) 787-5181

Dr. Earl Mindell's

What You Should Know About Creating Your Personal Vitamin Plan

PART I
Getting Acquainted with Your Supplements

CHAPTER 1

The ABC's of Supplements

Entering a store that specializes in selling supplements can be an overwhelming experience for someone who doesn't know their ABC's—that's vitamin A, vitamin B and vitamin C! This book is designed to give you a basic overview of what I consider to be your essential daily supplements, including vitamins, minerals, amino acids and antioxidants. You'll also find individual vitamin plans for your age, sex and lifestyle, as well as plenty of information about treating specific health concerns with nutritional supplements.

You'll notice that all of the supplement amounts I recommend are higher than the RDA (Recommended Dietary Allowance) set by the government. This is because the RDA is the amount of the vitamin you need to take to keep you from getting a vitamin deficiency disease. This is a long way from the amount of vitamins you need to keep you in great health for the rest of your life!

If you start with my basic vitamin plan and adapt to your own personal needs, you'll be well on your way to a life of optimal health and energy. For more details on any of the topics in this book, you can refer to the long list of other books I've written in the back of this book.

DO I REALLY NEED TO TAKE VITAMINS?

If you were to eat the best possible diet of nutrient-rich organic foods, and live a stress-free life, and your

90

environment was free of pollutants and toxins, you would not need vitamins. The reality of our lives is much different. It is virtually impossible to escape the pervasive pollution of our environment. Our soil is depleted of many essential minerals, and by the time once-fresh fruits and vegetables reach us in the supermarket, they have lost much of their nutritional value. We eat processed foods and junk foods with little or no nutritional value, and we eat dozens of pounds of sugar and salt per year more than is good for us. Add to that the stresses of daily life, prescription drugs, exposure to estrogenic hormones in meat, and all the other factors in our daily lives that pull our biochemistry out of balance, and the need for vitamins becomes apparent. In today's world, we need to take supplements just to maintain our health and prevent the onset of chronic diseases.

Taking vitamins and other supplements is health insurance that makes up for what you're not getting in your diet, and for the added nutritional demands made on the body by stressful lifestyles. Illness, aging and genetic weaknesses add to your individual nutritional needs. If there is a lot of cancer in your immediate family, you should be taking the supplements that are known to help prevent cancer, such as vitamin E and selenium. If your family has a history of heart disease, you need to create a heart-healthy lifestyle that includes a low-fat diet, plenty of exercise, and plenty of antioxidants and magnesium.

The key to creating your own individual vitamin plan is paying attention to your body's needs. If you find you're getting colds a lot, there are lifestyle factors you'll want to evaluate, such as whether you're getting enough sleep, whether you're allergic to something in your diet or something in your home or office, or maybe simply whether you're dressing warmly enough in cold weather. But you'll also want to increase your vitamin C consumption, your vitamin E consumption, and possibly your zinc (and you may want to take the useful herb echinacea) at the first sign of the sniffles.

Taking vitamins is not a substitute for a good diet or a healthy lifestyle. A vitamin can never reproduce all the nutrition packed into a fresh vegetable, or an egg, for example. The single biggest factor that shows up in studies of heart disease, cancer and aging over and over again, is that those who eat the most fresh vegetables live the longest, healthiest lives. And no amount of antioxidants will substitute for drinking plenty of clean water and moderate exercise. Nonetheless, taking vitamins is your backup plan for good health, providing the extra support you need to go beyond simply maintaining your health to having lots of energy and a clear mind.

FOR BEST RESULTS . . .

Most vitamins and minerals are best absorbed when taken with other foods, spaced out as evenly as possible during the day. The best time to take supplements is after meals. The amino acids are an exception to this. If you are taking a separate amino acid supplement, it is usually best to take it between meals.

Since some vitamins can be excreted in the urine, taking your vitamins after breakfast, after lunch and after dinner will give you the highest body level of nutrients. If you must take your vitamins all at one time, taking them after the largest meal of the day will usually give the best results.

Minerals and vitamins are mutually dependent upon each other for proper absorption. For example, vitamin C aids in the absorption of iron. Calcium aids in the absorption of vitamin D, and zinc aids in the absorption of vitamin A. So take your minerals and vitamins together.

TABLETS, CAPSULES AND LIQUIDS

Supplements come in many forms, but the most common are tablets, capsules and liquids. Multivitamins generally come in tablet form, but be sure they aren't so large you can't swallow them, and that they actually dissolve once they get to your digestive system. One way to find out how well vitamin tablets dissolve is to drop one in a little bit of vinegar, which approximates the acidity of your stomach. Depending on its size, the tablet should be nearly completely dissolved within an hour. If it isn't, you can bet you're not getting the full value from it. Some supplements work best in the small intestine, and these may be put into a tablet with a special coating that doesn't allow it to dissolve until it is out of the stomach.

Capsules are usually gelatin shells filled with the powdered form of the supplement. The gelatin dissolves quickly in the stomach, allowing the supplement to begin its work right away.

If you have trouble absorbing nutrients, you may want to consider some of the powdered or liquid vitamins, which don't have to be broken down as much in the gut.

CHAPTER 2

Vitamins Everyone Should Take Every Day

There are some vitamins that everyone, regardless of age or lifestyle, should take every day. These vitamins are essential for good health and peak energy, as they have a great many jobs to do in the body.

VITAMIN A / BETA-CAROTENE

Vitamin A is a fat-soluble vitamin that is stored in your body and doesn't need to be supplemented daily except in relatively small amounts. In fact, taking vitamin A in large doses over a long period of time can cause a toxic reaction because it accumulates in the body.

Vitamin A promotes growth, strong bones, healthy skin, is essential to the production of sex hormones, and works closely with zinc. People with acne can often eradicate it just by taking a vitamin A supplement for a few months. Vitamin A is also known as an anti-infective because it can help fight infections. In fact, if you have any type of lung infection, taking an extra vitamin A supplement for a week or two can help knock it out. Vitamin A is also called the ophthalmic vitamin because it helps improve eyesight.

Vitamin A is found in many vegetables, especially the orange and yellow vegetables such as carrots, squash, yams and cantaloupe. It's also found in liver, fish oil and eggs. One carrot can deliver up to 15,000

International Units of beta-carotene. Add a carrot a day to your apple a day!

Beta-carotene is a precursor to vitamin A, meaning that the body can make vitamin A from beta-carotene. That's the best way to get your vitamin A in a supplement, because it doesn't accumulate in the body the way vitamin A does. Beta-carotene is a potent antioxidant. Many recent studies have shown that people who have plenty of beta-carotene in their diet have a lower rate of cancer and coronary artery disease.

THE B-COMPLEX VITAMINS

The B-complex family are water-soluble vitamins involved in nearly every function of the body, from the manufacture of sex hormones and the health of brain neurons, to breaking down food and forming healthy red blood cells. The B vitamins play a key role in converting carbohydrate foods into glucose, or simple sugars, for use as energy.

The B-complex vitamins I'm going to cover here include vitamin B_1 (thiamine), vitamin B_2 (riboflavin), vitamin B_3 (niacin), vitamin B_6 (pyridoxine), vitamin B_{12} (cyanocobalamin), biotin, folic acid, inositol and vitamin B_5 (calcium pantothenate). It's best to take the B-complex vitamins together, because too much or too little of one can throw the others out of balance.

The B vitamins are found in whole grains, many nuts and root vegetables, meat, poultry, fish, eggs, dairy products and fruit.

VITAMIN B₁/Thiamine

Vitamin B_1 promotes growth, aids in the digestion of carbohydrates, can improve your mental attitude, can help fight sea and air sickness, relieves dental postoperative pain, and aids in the treatment of shingles and other herpes viruses. Vitamin B_1 is also essential for normal functioning of nerve tissues, muscles and heart. Taking vitamin B_1 as a supplement can create an odor on the skin that humans can't smell, but that repels insects, especially mosquitoes.

Smokers, drinkers, heavy sugar consumers, antacid users and those on birth control pills need more B_1.

Vitamin B_1 can cause high blood pressure in excess.

VITAMIN B_2/Riboflavin

Vitamin B_2 aids in growth and reproduction, promotes healthy hair, skin and nails, alleviates eye fatigue, eliminates sore mouth and lips, helps your body burn carbohydrates, fats and proteins. A deficiency of vitamin B_2 may cause a decreased ability to generate antibodies, which help the body resist disease. A deficiency may also result in itching and burning of the eyes, cracking of the corners of the lips, and inflammation of the mouth. If you are a heavy coffee or alcohol drinker, on the Pill, under a lot of stress, or eat lots of processed foods (please don't!), you may need extra vitamin B_2. Natural sources of vitamin B_2 include liver, kidney, milk, cheese, and most B_1 sources.

VITAMIN B_3/Niacin/niacinamide

Niacin is the most potent and effective cholesterol-lowering substance known. The only reason it isn't the best-selling cholesterol-lowering medicine is because it's an inexpensive, natural substance that can't be patented by the drug companies. If they can't patent it, they can't charge you high prices, so they aren't interested in promoting it. Niacin not only lowers LDL or "bad" cholesterol, it also raises HDL or "good" cholesterol. (If your physician has you on cholesterol-lowering drugs, don't stop taking them without supervision.)

Niacin has gotten some bad press. Some forms of it can cause flushing and itching, and high prolonged doses of timed-release niacin can cause liver problems. If you begin with a small dose and gradually work your way up to a higher dose, you should be able to minimize these problems. Niacinamide is more often used than niacin, since it minimizes the burning, flushing and itching of the skin that frequently occurs with nicotinic acid. More recently, some vitamin manufacturers have developed "no-flush" niacin formulas that deliver all of the benefits of niacin without the unpleasant side effects. These formulas are made by combining niacin with inositol hexanicotinate, an ester involved in sending messages within the nervous system. In any case, niacin is still safer and more effective than any of the pharmaceutical cholesterol-lowering drugs.

Niacin also aids in promoting a healthy digestive system, gives you healthy skin, can prevent or ease the severity of migraine headaches, increases circulation, especially in the upper body, can reduce high blood pressure, is an antidiarrheal, increases your energy through proper food utilization, helps fight canker sores, helps fight bad breath, is a possible cancer inhibitor, and is necessary for the metabolism of sugar.

Niacin is found naturally in lean meat, whole grains, green vegetables, and beans.

VITAMIN B₆/Pyridoxine

This vitamin is actually a group of vitamins called pyridoxine, pyridoxal and pyridoxamine, but B₆ is often just called pyridoxine. This important vitamin is crucial to the formation of all the steroid hormones, including the sex hormones and the cortisones. Women can often correct PMS and menopause problems simply by taking a vitamin B₆ supplement. It also helps protect against osteoporosis. This B vitamin also plays an essential role in maintaining a healthy nervous system and a healthy cardiovascular system. Researchers have recently recognized that a high level of homocysteine, a by-product of amino acid metabolism, is at least as important a risk factor in heart disease as high cholesterol or high blood pressure, and vitamin B_6, together with the B vitamins folic acid and vitamin B_{12}, reduces the level of homocysteine in the body.

Vitamin B_6 also helps assimilate protein and fat, aids in converting tryptophan to niacin, is an antinauseant (effective for morning sickness), can help with PMS and menopause symptoms, helps synthesize antiaging nucleic acids, reduces "cotton mouth" and urination problems caused by tricyclic antidepressant drugs, reduces night muscle spasms, leg cramps and hand numbness, and works as a natural diuretic. If you want to know more about vitamin B_6, I highly recommend Dr. Alan Gaby's book on the subject, *The Doctor's Guide to Vitamin B_6* (Rodale Press, 1984).

Vitamin B_6 occurs naturally in meat, fish, egg yolk, cantaloupe, cabbage, milk, soy products, peanuts, and brown rice.

A deficiency of vitamin B_6 may result in nervousness, insomnia, skin eruptions and loss of muscular control.

Vitamin B_6 can be toxic in high doses. Please don't take over 500 mg a day.

VITAMIN B_{12}/Cobalamin

Vitamin B_{12} is commonly known as the "red vitamin," cobalamin. Since it is so effective in small doses, it is one of the few vitamins generally recommended in microgram (mcg) doses. Vitamin B_{12} is not well absorbed in the digestive tract, so the best ways to take it in are intranasally or sublingually (under the tongue).

I believe that a very high percentage of senility

symptoms in older people are caused by a simple vitamin B_{12} and folic acid deficiency. As we age, we don't produce as much stomach acid and as a result we don't absorb our food as well. This is particularly true of the B vitamins, and especially B_{12}. Many older people tend to have poor nutrition anyway, but even with good nutrition, if there is an absorption problem, a vitamin B_{12} deficiency may result. Anyone over the age of 50 who is experiencing problems such as memory loss, forgetfulness, depression, loss of appetite, and fatigue, should try a few weeks of B_{12} shots (given by doctors and other health care professionals) to see if the symptoms clear up. Supplements of folic acid and vitamin B_6 should be given along with the B_{12}, as they work best together.

Vitamin B_{12} also forms and regenerates red blood cells which carry oxygen to the tissues, giving you more energy and preventing anemia, promotes growth and gives children an increased appetite, is important for maintenance of a healthy nervous system, can relieve irritability, improves circulation, memory, and balance, and can enhance immunity in the elderly. Vitamin B_{12} also plays an important role, along with folic acid and vitamin B_6, in keeping homocysteine levels low. As I mentioned earlier, homocysteine raises the risk of heart disease.

Vitamin B_{12} is found naturally in liver, beef, pork, eggs, milk, cheese. Vitamin B_{12} is only found in animal foods in significant amounts, so if you are a vegetarian it is important to take a B_{12} supplement.

BIOTIN

Biotin is one of the more recently discovered B vitamins, but it is a key vitamin in maintaining healthy hair and skin. It can keep your hair from turning gray, prevent baldness, ease muscle pains, and is important for healthy skin.

Biotin is found naturally in whole grains, milk, vegetables and nuts. It is present in minute quantities in every living cell and is also synthesized by intestinal bacteria.

A deficiency of biotin may lead to hair loss, extreme exhaustion, drowsiness, muscle pains and loss of appetite.

CHOLINE

Choline is an ingredient in lecithin, a naturally-occurring fat emulsifier found in eggs, soy and other legumes, nuts and some meats such as liver. Choline is one of the few substances able to penetrate the blood-brain barrier, going directly to brain cells, where it plays a role in transmitting nerve impulses. For this reason, taking lecithin may help with memory, ability to learn, symptoms of senility and Alzheimer's.

Because of its effects on fats, choline can lower cholesterol, aids the liver in removing poisons and drugs from your bloodstream, is necessary for normal fat metabolism, and minimizes excessive deposits of fat in liver.

Lecithin and choline are found naturally in egg yolks, green leafy vegetables and legumes.

A deficiency of choline may result in cirrhosis and fatty degeneration of the liver, and hardening of the arteries.

FOLIC ACID

Folic acid has recently been recognized as a key vitamin in preventing a type of birth defect called neural tube defects, such as spina bifida. It is important that all sexually active women at any risk whatsoever for getting pregnant get at least 200 mcg of folic acid every day, and preferably 400 mcg.

Folic acid also works hand in hand with vitamin B_6 and vitamin B_{12} to reduce the levels of harmful homocysteine in the blood. A deficiency of folic acid, vitamin B_6 and vitamin B_{12} significantly raises your risk of heart disease by raising homocysteine levels.

Folic acid also improves lactation in nursing women, can act as a pain reliever, delays gray hair (along with PABA and pantothenic acid), prevents canker sores, helps against anemia (along with iron, copper and vitamin C), is essential to the formation of red blood cells by its action on the bone marrow, aids in protein metabolism, and contributes to normal growth.

Too much folic acid can cause problems for epileptics and people with allergies.

Folic acid is found naturally in deep green leafy vegetables, and meat.

INOSITOL

Inositol combines with choline to form lecithin, and has many of the same benefits. It can be very helpful in treating eczema. It also lowers cholesterol, is important for healthy hair, helps metabolize body fat, is a relaxant, and can help relieve diabetic peripheral neuropathy.

Inositol is found naturally in fruits, nuts, whole grains, milk, and meat. Cantaloupe and citrus fruits are especially good sources.

VITAMIN B_5/Calcium Pantothenate

Calcium pantothenate is also called pantothenic acid. It is involved in the growth of cells, helps maintain normal skin, is crucial to the development of the central nervous system, is required for synthesis of antibodies, is necessary for normal digestive processes, helps heal wounds, prevents fatigue, is an antiallergy and stress supplement, and fights infections. In some people calcium pantothenate helps relieve arthritis symptoms, but in other people it can aggravate them.

Calcium pantothenate is found naturally in organ meats, eggs, whole grains, bran, peas.

VITAMIN C

Vitamin C, also called ascorbic acid, is water-soluble, and one of the superstars of the vitamin world. It is a powerful antioxidant that slows the aging process and helps prevent heart disease and cancer. It also plays an important role in healing wounds, helps prevent fatigue, is an antihistamine, helping to reduce allergy symptoms, helps fight infections by building antibodies, can stop bleeding gums, lowers cholesterol, is an anticancer agent, prevents the production of nitrosamines (cancer-causing agents), is a natural laxative, lowers the incidence of blood clots in the veins, therefore decreasing the risk of heart attack and stroke, decreases the severity and length of the common cold, and increases the absorption of iron. Vitamin C works as a team with other vitamins, minerals and enzymes, strengthening the collagen in connective tissue and promoting capillary integrity.

Vitamin C is found naturally in nearly all fresh foods and meat. It is especially high in citrus fruits, berries, greens, cabbages and peppers. Vitamin C is destroyed by cooking, which is one of the many reasons it is important to eat plenty of fresh, raw fruits and vegetables.

Vitamin C in large doses can cause mild diarrhea. Either buy an esterfied form of vitamin C, or back off the dose until the diarrhea stops.

VITAMIN D

Vitamin D is also called calciferous, ergosterol, and the "sunshine vitamin." This hormonelike vitamin regulates the use of calcium and phosphorus in the body and is therefore necessary for the proper formation of teeth and bones. It is especially important in infancy and childhood. Most of our vitamin D is manufactured in the body when our skin is exposed to sunlight. This is why it's important to get regular sun. Taken with A and C, vitamin D can help to prevent colds. It is also used to treat conjunctivitis.

Vitamin D is also found naturally in fish oil, fat, and dairy products. Vitamin D should not be taken in high doses long term because it accumulates in the body and can be toxic at high doses. However, it can be an essential vitamin for people who aren't getting outdoors in the sun.

VITAMIN E

Vitamin E is also called tocopherol. It is available in several different forms, both as a liquid and solid. Vitamin E is another superstar in the vitamin world, able to help us fend off heart disease and important to hundreds of biochemical processes in the body. Vitamin E is a powerful antioxidant that slows the aging process and also helps prevent cancer. It works with beta-carotene to protect the lungs from pollution, prevents and dissolves blood clots, helps prevent scarring when used externally on the skin, accelerates burn healing, can lower blood pressure by its diuretic action, prevents night cramps, lazy leg and leg cramps, helps prevent cataracts, and enhances the immune system.

Vitamin E is found naturally in whole grains,

green leafy vegetables, vegetable oils, meat, eggs, and avocados.

Today many cardiologists recommend 400 IU of Vitamin E daily. The dry (succinate) form of Vitamin E is preferred for people over 40 because it is more easily absorbed by the digestive system.

BIOFLAVONOIDS

Bioflavonoids are organic compounds found in plants. These powerful substances reduce inflammation and pain, strengthen blood vessels, improve circulation, fight bacteria and viruses, improve liver function, lower cholesterol levels and improve vision. Bioflavonoids help prevent bruising by strengthening capillary walls. For this reason, they are also helpful for diabetics in improving circulation, and can help prevent eye problems such as cataracts and macular degeneration. Bioflavonoids are also beneficial in hypertension, and help build resistance to infections and colds.

Vitamin C is found combined with bioflavonoids in nature, and in supplements works much more effectively when combined with bioflavonoids.

Bioflavonoids are found in a wide variety of plants. Some of the best food sources are the white material underneath citrus fruit peels, peppers, and berries. Although bioflavonoids are not considered essential to life, and therefore are not classified as vitamins, it is becoming clear that they *are* essential to good health.

Whatever vitamin C you are taking should be combined with a bioflavonoid complex. Each works best when combined with the other.

CHAPTER 3

Minerals Everyone Should Take Every Day

Minerals work in partnership with hormones, enzymes, amino acids and vitamins. They are required to build and maintain the structure of the body. They are involved in the breakdown of food during digestion, and some are instrumental in maintaining fluid balance inside cells. Those that are currently considered essential for human nutrition are: calcium, phosphorus, iron, potassium, selenium, magnesium and zinc. In reality however, many more minerals are needed to maintain optimal health. Chromium, cobalt, copper, manganese and potassium are important in their own right, even though we only require them in very small amounts.

Processed or refined foods (for example: white flour and white sugar) are almost devoid of minerals, which is one reason I strongly recommend eating whole foods such as grains, fruits and vegetables, which are very rich in minerals in their unrefined state.

Another reason we tend to be deficient in minerals is that our soil is depleted. Modern agricultural methods using commercial fertilizers do not replace the rich array of minerals found naturally in soil, so vegetables grown in those soils do not have the minerals we need for good health. This is one of the best reasons I know of to eat organic fruits and vegetables (besides reducing your exposure to pesticides).

Unless you are trying to correct a specific nutritional deficiency under the supervision of a health-care professional, minerals should only be taken in the recommended doses. An excess of minerals can cause just as many problems as a deficiency.

Let's take a closer look at the minerals you should be getting in your daily vitamin program.

CALCIUM

Calcium is the most abundant mineral in the body. It builds and maintains bones and teeth, helps blood to clot, aids vitality and endurance, regulates heart rhythm and helps muscles relax. Calcium also plays a role in maintaining fluid balance within the cells. Calcium can't do its work maintaining strong bones without its partners magnesium and phosphorus. Most of us get plenty of phosphorus in our diets, but many North Americans are deficient in magnesium, and calcium should always be taken with magnesium. There is some disagreement about what the ratio of calcium to magnesium should be, but most supplements provide a three to one ratio of calcium to magnesium, which is fine. Because of their relaxing effect on the muscles, calcium and magnesium can be taken just before bed to aid in sleeping and to prevent leg cramps.

Contrary to popular opinion, milk is not a good source of calcium because it has a poor calcium-to-magnesium ratio, so the body can't put it to work. I believe dairy products cause more health problems than they solve, and I recommend that you get the majority of your calcium from fresh vegetables, especially leafy green vegetables, soy foods, sardines, salmon and nuts. A high protein diet and excessive consumption of phosphorus-containing sodas can deplete calcium from the bones.

BORON

Boron is a trace mineral that helps retard bone loss and works with calcium, magnesium and vitamin D to help prevent osteoporosis (brittle bones). Boron is abundant in apples and grapes.

CHROMIUM

Chromium works with insulin in the metabolism of sugar and helps the body utilize protein and fats. Taken in conjunction with exercise, chromium helps the body burn off fat more efficiently. It is best to take chromium in the form of chromium picolinate. Chromium also helps prevent and lower high blood pressure.

COBALT

Cobalt is a stimulant to the production of red blood cells, is a component of vitamin B_{12}, and is necessary for normal growth. A deficiency of cobalt can cause anemia.

COPPER

Copper and zinc balance each other in the body, and a deficiency of one can cause an excess of the other. Copper is necessary for absorption and utilization of iron and the formation of red blood cells.

IRON

Iron is required in manufacture of hemoglobin, a component of blood, and helps carry oxygen in the blood. It works with many enzymes in biochemical reactions in the body, and to be used efficiently must also have copper, cobalt, manganese and vitamin C.

Iron is not efficiently excreted from the body, and can accumulate in tissues. Recent research has shown that excessive amounts of iron in the tissues raise the risk of heart disease. Some researchers theorize that part of the reason a woman's risk of heart disease increases after menopause is that she is not losing iron every month during menstruation. Although iron is an essential mineral, it is important not to take too much iron in supplement form. A deficiency can cause a specific disease called iron deficiency anemia.

MAGNESIUM

Magnesium is one of the superstars of the mineral world. It is necessary for calcium and vitamin C metabolism and literally hundreds of enzyme reactions in the body. It plays a key role in regulating fluid balance in the cells, and is essential for normal functioning of the nervous, muscular and cardiovascular systems. Magnesium deficiency is very common in North America, and I believe that it is a more common and important risk factor for heart disease than mainstream medicine acknowledges. I recommend that anyone with heart disease or at risk for heart disease take an extra supplement of 300-400 mg of magnesium daily. Fatigue and muscle weakness can also be signs of magnesium deficiency.

Magnesium is found naturally in whole grains, figs, nuts and seeds, bananas and other fruits, and green vegetables.

MANGANESE

Manganese is an important trace mineral that activates various enzymes and other minerals and is related to proper utilization of vitamins B_1 and E. Manganese is also involved with thyroid function, the central nervous system and digestion.

POTASSIUM

Potassium is a key mineral in regulating the pH balance and fluid balance in the body. It balances sodium in the cells and, along with calcium and magnesium, regulates heart rhythm. Potassium can be depleted by any type of abnormally large fluid loss such as strenuous exercise, diarrhea, hypoglycemia, and the use of diuretics such as those used to lower blood pressure. When potassium is deficient, it can cause nerve and muscle dysfunction, bloating due to water retention, ringing in the ears, and insomnia. Potassium is naturally found in citrus fruits, cantaloupe, tomatoes, watercress, all green leafy vegetables, the mints, sunflower seeds, bananas and potatoes. Most people can easily get enough potassium in their daily diet, but many multivitamins contain potassium. Please don't take potassium supplements without the supervision of a health care professional, as an excess can throw other minerals out of balance and affect fluid balance in the cells.

SELENIUM

Selenium could be called the anticancer mineral. Over and over again population studies have shown that people living in geographical areas containing plenty of selenium in the soil have lower rates of cancer, and those living in areas with selenium-depleted soil have a higher rate of cancer, especially colon cancer. Selenium is an antioxidant that also stimulates the immune system. It works synergistically with vitamin E, each enhancing the actions of the other. Selenium is found in high concentrations in semen, and men seem to need more of this mineral than women. A selenium deficiency can cause dandruff, dry skin and fatigue.

ZINC

An essential mineral, zinc plays multiple roles. It controls muscle contractions, along with magnesium and calcium, helps normal tissue function, and is essential in protein and carbohydrate metabolism and the functioning of the immune system. A lack of zinc in your diet can increase fatigue and cause a susceptibility to infection and injury, as well as a reduction in alertness. When you exercise vigorously, you lose a lot of zinc, so it's important for athletes to take a zinc supplement. Zinc is found in many foods, including most vegetables, whole grains, dairy products, many nuts and seeds, fish and meat.

Zinc should be present in all good multivitamin formulas. But as with all minerals, please don't take zinc in excess, as it will cause other imbalances in your body. Zinc works best in combination with vitamin A, calcium and phosphorus.

CHAPTER 4

The Amazing Amino Acids

Protein is made up of amino acids. Although there are dozens of amino acids, only some amino acids are produced in the body. All eight of the essential amino acids are made in very small amounts by the bacteria found in the intestines, but they must also be supplied from food intake.

THE ESSENTIAL AMINO ACIDS

Lysine	Phenylalanine
Leucine	Threonine
Isoleucine	Tryptophan
Methionine	Valine

The following amino acids are essential for pregnant women for their developing fetus, and for infants: histidine, taurine and cysteine. Eric R. Braverman and Carl C. Pfeiffer, in their book *The Healing Nutrients Within*, state the following amino acids to be conditionally essential, and necessary for anyone under stress: alanine, arginine, aspartic acid, carnitine, cystine, GABA, glutamic acid, glutamine, glycine, homocysteine (toxic in high doses), hydroxyproline, proline, and serine.

Amino acids play a variety of important roles in every part of the body, including the immune system, the digestive system, metabolism, detoxification, and glucose balance. In the brain, some of the amino acids taken as supplements work very well to combat depression, enhance mood and improve sleep, while others improve memory and cognitive abilities.

When we eat proteins, they are broken down into proteins or peptides, which are proteins made of only a few amino acids, and then absorbed into the body.

TAKING AMINO ACIDS

All amino acids should be taken between meals with juice or water, and not with protein, unless they are included in a multivitamin. Since individual amino acids can have such a powerful effect on the body, I recommend that, if you're taking them to treat a specific chronic problem such as heart disease or depression, you work with a health care professional.

Many amino acids serve as precursors for others. For example, cysteine is a precursor to glutathione, and since glutathione is somewhat unstable in supplement form, you can take cysteine or N-acetyl cysteine as a supplement to boost your glutathione levels.

If you're taking amino acids, taking a B-vitamin complex at the same time will enhance their absorption and metabolism.

Here is a complete list of all of the amino acids, grouped by their molecular structure and function in the body, as delineated by Braverman and Pfeiffer. If you want to know more about amino acids, I highly recommend their book.

Aromatic amino acids
Phenylalanine
Tyrosine
Tryptophan

Sulfur amino Acids
Cysteine and Glutathione
Taurine

Methionine
Homocysteine

Urea cycle amino acids
Arginine and citrulline
Ornithine

Glutamate amino acids
Glutamic acid, GABA and glutamine
Proline and hydroxyproline
Aspartic acid–asparagine

Threonine amino acids
Threonine
Glycine
Serine
Alanine

Branched chain amino acids
Leucine, isoleucine and valine

Amino acids with important metabolites
Lysine
Carnitine
Histidine

Here are some of the amino acids that should be included in vitamin regimens, especially if you are a vegetarian, aren't absorbing nutrients well, have problems with depression, or simply need a high-powered vitamin regimen:

ALANINE

Alanine is a nonessential amino acid that enhances the immune system, lowers the risk of kidney stones, and aids in alleviating hypoglycemia by regulating sugar. Alanine is released by the muscles for energy, and athletes may enhance their performance by taking alanine supplements. In very high doses alanine suppresses taurine. Alanine has also been used successfully to treat epilepsy, high cholesterol, and liver disease in alcoholics.

ARGININE

Arginine is a conditionally essential amino acid that increases sperm count in men, accelerates wound healing, tones muscle tissue, helps metabolize stored body fat, and promotes physical and mental alertness. Arginine is important in estrogen production, and a deficiency may contribute to an estrogen deficiency. Research with rodents has demonstrated that arginine can reduce the growth of tumors. Arginine can aggravate herpes and bring on an outbreak. Those who suffer from herpes outbreaks should avoid arginine supplements and arginine-containing foods such as nuts, chocolate and coffee. Arginine also should not be taken by growing children.

ASPARTIC ACID

Aspartic acid is a nonessential amino acid that is highly concentrated in the body. It can enhance the immune system, as well as increase stamina and endurance. Aspartic acid should be used as a supplement with great care because it is one of the major excitatory neurotransmitters in the brain, and can be toxic in excess. The artificial sweetener aspartame breaks down in the stomach to aspartic acid and phenylalanine (among other things), and consuming excessive amounts of these amino acids in people who are sensitive to them is related to the widespread health problems caused by aspartame, including headaches, dizziness and seizures.

CARNITINE

Although carnitine is not an essential amino acid, a deficiency can cause fatigue, muscle weakness, heart disease, acidic blood, high triglyceride levels, and brain degeneration. Taking carnitine as a supplement can enhance the body's ability to burn fat, prevent heart disease and improve brain deterioration as we age.

Lysine is a precursor to carnitine, and to manufacture carnitine, the body also needs vitamin B_6, niacin, iron, and vitamin C.

If you're at risk for heart disease, or have heart disease, carnitine is an essential supplement for you. Carnitine supplements can lower triglyceride levels, raise HDL (good) cholesterol, lower LDL (bad) cholesterol, and it improves irregular heartbeats, reduces angina attacks and has an overall strengthening effect on the heart.

Carnitine is an especially important supplement to take when you're losing weight because it cleans up substances called ketones in the blood, formed when the body is breaking down fat.

While carnitine is being used successfully to treat the symptoms of Alzheimer's and senility, you don't need to have a failing memory to benefit from it. Studies have shown that carnitine supplementation improves long term memory, increases alertness and improves learning ability and can improve mood.

Carnitine's ability to protect brain neurons and enhance their responsiveness also makes it one of our most important anti-aging supplements. Carnitine essentially acts as an antioxidant in the brain.

The forms of carnitine I recommend are either L-carnitine, acetyl L-carnitine, or L-acetylcarnitine. Please do not take the synthetic D or DL forms of carnitine, as they can have negative side effects.

CYSTINE, CYSTEINE

Cysteine is another conditionally essential amino acid and an important antiaging nutrient. Cystine and cysteine can be readily converted by the body into one another. Cysteine's most important role in the body is detoxification. In addition, it is an antioxidant. Cysteine is a precursor to the important amino acids taurine and glutathione.

When given as a supplement, cysteine raises glutathione levels in the body. Because of this, it is used routinely in hospital emergency rooms to prevent liver damage when people overdose on drugs or alcohol; to detoxify in cases of heavy metal poisoning, and is used to protect against the harmful side effects of chemotherapy and radiation. Cysteine is currently being used successfully to raise T-cell levels in AIDS patients. Cysteine is also important in preventing eye problems such as cataracts and macular degeneration.

Foods that contain high levels of cysteine include onions, garlic, yogurt, wheat germ and red meat.

A form of cysteine called N-acetyl cysteine is widely used in Europe for coughs, asthma prevention and chronic bronchitis, because it is very effective at breaking up mucus in the lungs. If you have a tendency to get a winter cough, take it at the first sign of lung troubles.

Please don't take more than the recommended dosage of cysteine, as an excess can upset the balance of your body's chemistry just as much as a deficiency can.

GAMMA-AMINOBUTYRIC ACID (GABA)

One of the best known substances that transmit nerve impulses to the brain (neurotransmitter), GABA has a calming effect. In the brain GABA balances glutamic acid, an excitatory amino acid. The three amino acids GABA, glutamic acid and glutamine are constantly being transformed into each other as needed by the body.

GABA plays a major role in brain function. The benzodiazepine drugs such as Valium work because they stimulate GABA receptors in the brain.

GABA optimizes the body's use of vitamin C, it can lower blood pressure, and it may be involved with the release of growth hormone.

GLUTAMIC ACID

Glutamic acid works closely with GABA, particularly in the brain. However, while GABA is calming, glutamic acid is the opposite, an excitatory brain amino acid. In people who are deficient in it, glutamic acid can help improve brain function, alleviate fatigue, and elevate mood. However, in excess glutamic acid can become an excitotoxin, overstimulating brain cells and killing them. I recommend you work with a healthcare professional when using glutamic acid as a supplement.

GLUTAMINE

Glutamine is the third in the trio of GABA and glutamic acid. It is abundant in the brain, and in the intestines, where it plays an important role in maintaining a healthy mucous lining. Taking glutamine before and after surgery can significantly reduce healing time. Manganese is a mineral that is essential to the synthesis of glutamine, and glutamine is essential to the synthesis of niacin, as is tryptophan. Glutamine has been used successfully to help alcoholics in the withdrawal process and can greatly decrease the craving for alcohol.

Glutamine seems to be a food for cancer tumors, so please don't take this as a supplement if you have cancer. Since it plays a role in regulating brain neurotransmitters, it can be toxic in high doses.

GLUTATHIONE

I call glutathione (known as GSH) the "triple threat" amino acid because it is a tripeptide made from the amino acids cysteine, glycine and glutamic acid. It is found in the cells of nearly all living organisms on earth, and its primary job is waste disposal. GSH has three main detox jobs in the body: 1) When there are free radicals lurking about, threatening to start an oxidation reaction, GSH catches them, neutralizes them, passes them on (often to another antioxidant such as vitamin E), and begins the cycle anew; 2) in the liver, GSH latches on to toxic substances and binds to them, so the liver can excrete them without being damaged; and 3) GSH prevents red blood cells from being damaged by neutralizing unstable forms of oxygen.

GSH also plays a role in fighting cancer, stabilizing blood sugar, and cellular repair after a stroke. Glutathione's antioxidant work is the front line defense for preventing oxidation of LDL cholesterol which damages the arteries. It's also crucial in protecting the lymphatic system and the digestive system from an overload of unstable lipids (fats and oils). If glutathione levels drop anywhere in the body, the burden of toxic stress goes up.

GSH is one of the most abundant substances in the body, and as long as we have a good supply of its building block cysteine (glycine and glutamic acid are rarely in short supply) and its cofactor selenium, it will be hard at work doing its detoxifying chores. GSH levels drop as we age, and can be depleted by an overload of rancid oils (such as polyunsaturated and partially hydrogenated vegetable oils), overexposure to poisons such as pesticides, and pharmaceutical drugs that stress the liver such as acetaminophen (Tylenol) and aspirin. Since glutathione often passes off its neutralized waste products to antioxidants such as vitamin C and vitamin E, a deficiency of these vitamins can impair its function.

If you have heart disease, are at a high risk for it, or have high LDL cholesterol levels, I recommend you try raising your glutathione· levels. The best way to raise glutathione levels is by taking a cysteine supplement. Once again, please stick to the recommended dosage; an excess of cysteine can cause as many problems as it solves.

GLYCINE

Glycine is a conditionally essential amino acid that produces glycogen which mobilizes glucose (blood sugar) from the liver, and bolsters the immune system. Like GABA and taurine, glycine has a calming effect on the brain. A deficiency is thought to be involved with Parkinson's disease, and it may increase acetylcholine in the brain, improving memory and cognitive function.

Glycine has a sweet taste that can mask bitterness, and it is sometimes used as a sweetener. It is also used as a food additive to prevent the rancidity of fats and to act as an antioxidant. Glycine can lower cholesterol, heal gout, and speeds up wound healing. It stimulates growth hormone, and can aid in healing of a swollen and infected prostate.

HISTIDINE

Although histidine is not an essential amino acid for adults, it is an amino acid that is essential to growth, from fetal growth through infancy. It is a precursor of histamine, which stimulates inflammation in allergies.

A histadine deficiency is found in many arthritis patients, and supplementation sometimes helps. Histidine can help keep people from biting their nails, dilate blood vessels, alleviate symptoms of rheumatoid arthritis, alleviate stress, and can help increase libido. A histidine deficiency contributes to the development of cataracts. Because elevated histadine levels can cause mental problems, it is not recommended as a daily supplement for adults.

ISOLEUCINE, LEUCINE AND VALINE

Isoleucine, leucine and valine are essential amino acids known as branched chain amino acids (BCAAs). They are key ingredients in the body's ability to handle stress and produce energy. They are used by the muscles for energy, and are needed in hemoglobin formation. Taking the BCAAs as a supplement can speed healing after surgery, and may help build muscle. The BCAAs may also be brain transmitters and have some ability to relieve pain. Alcoholics and drug addicts tend to be deficient in leucine, glutamine, GABA and citrulline.

PHENYLALANINE

Phenylalanine is an essential amino acid that plays a key part in brain function and is a major precursor to many brain chemicals, including the amino acid tyrosine, and the catecholamines such as dopamine and epinephrine. Other brain chemicals such as vasopressin, somatostatin and ACTH contain phenylalanine. Morphine and codeine contain phenylalanine.

Like the other amino acids that affect brain function, phenylalanine can be very helpful as a supplement if it is deficient in some way, but can be harmful in excess. The artificial sweetener aspartame breaks down in the stomach to form aspartic acid and phenylalanine. The phenylalanine accounts for some of the adverse reactions to the sweetener. Some people are born with a sensitivity to phenylalanine called phenylketonuria (PKU). If not caught in infancy and foods containing phenylalanine avoided, PKU can cause serious retardation.

In people who are deficient in phenylalanine, it can improve memory and mental alertness, act as an antidepressant, help suppress appetite, reduce pain and increase sexual interest. It can also raise blood pressure, so be cautious in its use if you have high blood pressure. It cannot be metabolized if a person is deficient in vitamin C.

I recommend taking phenylalanine in the D or DL-phenylalanine form.

LYSINE

Lysine is an essential amino acid involved in metabolism, muscle tissue, the immune system, and growth. A deficiency may cause nausea, dizziness and anemia. Taking it as a supplement helps improve concentration, enhances fertility, aids in preventing fever blisters or cold sores (herpes simplex) and shortens the healing period for herpes. Lysine is found in meat, eggs, fish, milk and cheese. When treating a herpes outbreak, up to 5 grams (5,000 mg) a day may be taken.

METHIONINE

Methionine is an essential amino acid and plays an important role in metabolism. It is a lipotropic agent, meaning it reduces fat, particularly in the liver. It also protects the kidneys, aids in lowering cholesterol, is a natural chelating agent for heavy metals, and aids in maintaining beautiful skin. It also builds new bony tissue. A deficiency of methionine may lead to heart disease, fatty degeneration and cirrhosis of the liver.

It has been used to treat schizophrenia, Parkinson's and depression. Methionine can be found in sunflower seeds, meat, eggs, fish, milk and cheese.

PROLINE AND HYDROXYPROLINE

Proline and hydroxyproline are conditionally essential amino acids that aid in wound healing, and can help increase learning ability. These two amino acids are found in the highest amounts in the body's collagen tissue. Hydroxyproline is most important in bone and connective tissue. Proline is one of the amino acids that seems to stimulate tumor development, and people with cancer should not take it as a supplement. In fact, it is probably not necessary to supplement proline or hydroxyproline at all, as they tend to be in the body in abundance, and an excess can cause imbalances in other amino acids.

SERINE

Serine is a conditionally essential amino acid that is made from glycine and can also be made into glycine and cystine. It can help alleviate pain and produces cellular energy. An excess in the body or very high doses can cause psychosis. Serine is another amino acid that promotes tumor growth and should not be taken by anyone who has cancer. There is no need to supplement serine as our bodies tend to make what we need in abundance.

TAURINE

Taurine is an amino acid that is essential to infants but nonessential to adults. It is a very useful amino acid in treating some forms of epilepsy. It plays an important role in the heart, eyes, brain, gallbladder and blood vessels, particularly keeping fluids and mineral balance in cells stable, and stabilizing cell membranes. Taurine is an important supplement for anyone who has heart disease, but should be taken under the guidance of a health care professional if you are on heart disease drugs. Taurine is also important in stabilizing cell membranes in the brain, and is a neurotransmitter, and as such can have a calming effect. It can improve memory, and has been used to treat insomnia, anxiety and high blood pressure. The food additive MSG can reduce taurine levels. Since taurine can enhance the action of insulin, diabetics and hypoglycemics should use it with care.

THREONINE

Threonine is an essential amino acid that can be deficient in vegetarian diets. It is a precursor to the important amino acid glycine, which acts as a brain sedative. Threonine is essential to normal growth, helps prevent fatty buildup in the liver, is necessary for utilization of protein in the diet, stimulates the immune system, and has been used to treat manic depression and multiple sclerosis. A deficiency results in negative hydrogen balance in the body. Threonine levels decline with age, making them valuable antiaging supplements.

TRYPTOPHAN

Tryptophan is an essential amino acid with many valuable uses. It is a precursor to niacin, which prevents pellagra and mental deficiency. It plays a role in regulating sleep and is closely tied to the production of serotonin in the brain. A deficiency causes insomnia. It is useful as a relaxant and antianxiety agent as well.

Tryptophan was widely used as a sleep aid until a contaminated batch made in Japan reportedly killed 11 people. Unfortunately, in spite of the fact that uncontaminated tryptophan is entirely safe and is used in baby foods and nutritional powders for senior citizens, the FDA has pulled it off the market as a nutritional supplement as of this writing. Tryptophan was pulled off the market within weeks before the drug Prozac was approved by the FDA. It is interesting that the inexpensive, safe and effective tryptophan does essentially the same thing in the brain that Prozac does, without the side effects. The fact that tryptophan is not available in the US is purely political and has no basis in a lack of safety.

TYROSINE

Tyrosine is a nonessential amino acid that acts as a precursor to many other amino acids and brain chemicals. It is important in times of stress, and plays a part in maintaining a healthy thyroid gland. It also yields L-dopa, making it useful in the treatment of Parkinson's disease. It has an important role in stimulating and modifying brain activity, helps control drug resistant depression and anxiety, as well as helping amphetamine takers to reduce their dosage to minimal levels in a few weeks. It can also help cocaine addicts kick their habit, by helping to avert the depression, fatigue and extreme irritability which accompany withdrawal. It can worsen the symptoms of schizophrenia.

The artificial sweetener aspartame raises tyrosine levels in the brain, which may cause toxicity in sensitive people.

CHAPTER 5

A Few Important Antioxidants

Antioxidants are one of your best forms of health insurance, both against the modern maladies that plague so many of us, such as heart disease, cancer and diabetes, and against the diseases of aging, such as arthritis and digestive difficulties. There are hundreds and probably even thousands of antioxidants, most of them found naturally in plants, particularly fresh fruits and vegetables, but also in herbs. Antioxidants are also present to some degree in seafood, and in some animal foods.

Antioxidants neutralize the damage of oxidation by squelching free radicals. What does all that mean? We can think of oxidation as similar to what happens to metal when it rusts, or what happens to an apple when it turns brown. Have you ever prevented a cut-up apple from turning brown by squeezing some lemon juice on it? The vitamin C in the lemon juice is an antioxidant that is stopping the oxidation process. When meat spoils, or oil goes rancid, oxidation is in process.

An unstable oxygen molecule has a missing electron, creating what is called a free radical. These unstable oxygen molecules go to war in the body, grabbing onto other cells in their attempt to find another electron and stabilize. Every time a free radical stabilizes itself by attacking another cell, it leaves the cell it attacked damaged. That cell becomes unstable and in turn goes after another, creating a chain reaction. This is the process known as oxidation.

The damage free radicals do includes cell mutation, cardiovascular disease, cataracts, macular degeneration, arthritis, diseases affecting the brain, the kidneys, the lungs, the digestive system and the immune system. Free radicals are involved in the damage done by alcoholism, aging, radiation injury, iron overload, and diseases that affect the blood, such as strokes. Once the process of oxidation begins, it can be hard to stop, so your best health plan is to prevent it in the first place.

Our bodies naturally produce free radicals as part of our complex interaction with oxygen. In fact, free radicals act as enzymes and chemical messengers, and we couldn't live without them. It is when they become excessive that we begin to get sick. They have become a problem largely because of the polluted environment we live in, and our poor diets.

The ideal body, with ideal nutrition, in an ideal environment, would have the ability to counteract the free radicals it produces with the antioxidants it takes in and produces, and keep them under control. Heavy exercise produces free radicals, but it also has beneficial effects on the body that help counteract them.

Every day we encounter dozens of environmental causes of free radical production. The biggest culprits we know of are pollutants such as smog, toxins such as chlorine, herbicides and pesticides, radiation, some food additives, cigarette smoke, many prescription drugs, and rancid oil. Furthermore, most Americans eat relatively few fresh fruits and vegetables, one of our main natural sources of antioxidants. In a typical day, most of us run into more free radical-producing situations than our bodies can keep up with. This is why we need antioxidant supplements.

Let's take a quick look at some of my favorite antioxidants.

COENZYME Q10 (UBIQUINOL)

This versatile and powerful antioxidant is the superstar when it comes to fighting "bad" or LDL cholesterol. It works well in combination with vitamin E.

CoQ10 is a vital enzyme, or catalyst to the production of energy in our cells. Without it, our cells simply won't work. Its chemical name is *ubiquinone*—it is ubiquitous, or everywhere, where there is life. Its levels in the human body are highest in the heart and liver. When we are ill or stressed, and as we age, our bodies are less able to produce CoQ10.

CoQ10 helps regulate heart function. Many older people whose heart function has degenerated and who try CoQ10, report an almost immediate boost in their energy levels. People who suffer from angina report that the pain disappears and they can do some exercise. Studies have shown that people on heart medications can greatly reduce their dosage of medicine if it is combined with CoQ10.

CoQ10 can work powerfully to heal gum disease.

Food sources are mackerel, sardines, soybeans, peanuts and walnuts.

All CoQ10 is not created equal—the powder inside the capsules should be dark yellow.

SUPEROXIDE DISMUTASE (SOD)

Superoxide dismutase (SOD) is an enzyme that acts as a potent antioxidant, especially with skin tissue, and may be able to slow the aging process. SOD is destroyed in the stomach, so it needs to be used either as a cream or taken in an enteric coated capsule which passes through the stomach intact and dissolves in the intestines. SOD injections have been used successfully to treat scleroderma, a hardening of the skin. SOD with liposome is expensive, but if you have a stubborn skin problem it might be worth a try.

THE BIOFLAVONOID ANTIOXIDANTS

QUERCETIN

You should get to know this antioxidant, anticancer and antiallergy agent. This bioflavonoid may also have antiviral properties. Red and yellow onions are the best food sources of quercetin, though most fruits and vegetables contain some. You can also get it as a supplement.

PROANTHOCYANIDINS/PCOS/GRAPESEED EXTRACT

PCOs are another powerful free radical neutralizer that, like quercetin, are a bioflavonoid. Because PCOs are water soluble, the body is able to quickly and easily use them as an antioxidant. They also reduce inflammation, improve circulation, and improve the flexibility of connective tissues. Although proanthocyanidins are found in many fruits and vegetables, much of the supply is depleted by the time it gets to our stomachs. Most fruits and vegetables are grown in depleted soil, picked before they are ripened, sprayed with pesticides and fungicides, and stored for long periods of time.

PCOs can also be very effective in relieving allergy symptoms, because they inhibit the release of histamines.

GINKGO BILOBA

Ginkgo biloba has been used by the Chinese medicinally for at least 5,000 years. They prize ginkgo leaves for their ability to improve blood flow to the brain, open up congested lungs, and improve blood flow to the extremities. The leaves of this ancient tree provide a powerful antiaging aid, particularly in regard to improving brain function. It improves memory, learning and communication ability, as well as other symptoms of senility. It can also cure dizziness and improve balance.

Ginkgo is one of the best-selling medicines in Europe, sold to an estimated 10 million people every year. It has been the subject of over 300 scientific studies. GBE, a standardized ginkgo biloba extract, is a government-approved medicine in Germany and is covered by health insurance there.

Ginkgo's healing abilities have to do with improving circulation and improving the flow of oxygen to the brain and extremities. However, its spectrum of activities is wide, thanks to the wide variety of substances it contains, including flavonoids, terpenoids (ginkgolides, bilobalide), ginkgo heterosides, proanthocyanidins (PCO's) and organic acids.

Ginkgo is also useful for treating vision problems such as cataracts, macular degeneration, varicose veins, cold or numb feet and hands, ringing of the ears (tinnitus), leg cramps, and headaches. It improves cholesterol levels and improves circulation to the heart.

GREEN TEA

Green tea, the most popular of Asian drinks, turns out to be a potent antioxidant. The antioxidants specific to green tea are polyphenols, bioflavonoids that act as super antioxidants by neutralizing harmful fats and oils, lowering cholesterol and blood pressure, blocking cancer-triggering mechanisms, inhibiting bacteria and viruses, improving digestion, and protecting against ulcers and strokes. The specific type of polyphenol found in green tea is called a catechin.

Green tea comes from the same plants as black tea does, but is simply picked and dried without fermentation, allowing more of the original catechin content to remain intact. Oolong, a semi-fermented tea, falls in between black and green tea. Green tea contains 30-42 percent catechins, Oolong tea contains 8-20 percent catechins, and black tea contains 3-10 percent catechins.

CHAPTER 6

The Wonder of Enzymes

There isn't a cell in the body that functions without the help of enzymes. Enzymes are the magic ingredient that makes all of the other ingredients in the body work together. It is estimated that enzymes are facilitating 36 million biochemical reactions in the human body every minute. There are thousands of different enzymes at work, each with its own individual assignment.

Without the appropriate enzyme to bind to, vitamins are just so much organic matter, minerals are just so much inorganic matter, and even oxygen itself is just another molecule. Enzymes regulate all living matter, plants and animals alike. Take away enzymes and you no longer have something that is living.

We can also look at enzymes as the guide that shows the vitamin or mineral or fat the way into the cell. Without the introduction of the enzyme, the cell might never know the identity of the nutrient. Enzymes also speed up processes which might take much longer without their help, they build proteins that create tissue, remove toxins, help prevent the aging process within cells, and change nutrients into useful energy.

The enzymes that we know about are divided by what their purpose is in the body: they are called oxidoreductases, transferases, hydrolases, lyases, isomerases, and ligases. The digestive enzymes are the hydrolases, and these are the ones we will examine more closely.

We are born with enzymes already in our bodies, and we get some from food. However, enzymes are very sensitive to heat and processing, (including microwaving and pasteurizing) so they are not found in cooked or processed food. This means you need to get your enzymes from fresh, uncooked food such as raw fruit and vegetables, or from enzyme supplements.

Some enzyme experts believe that factors such as stress, malnutrition, junk food, alcohol and cigarettes destroy and thus deplete enzymes. They theorize that many digestive problems and immune disorders happen when we are deficient in enzymes.

Some of the best food sources of enzymes are avocados, bananas, papayas, mangoes, pineapples, sprouts and the aspergillus plant.

ENZYMES AND PAIN

There are new clinical studies showing that enzymes help reduce inflammation caused by arthritis, injuries to joints and other connective tissues such as muscle sprains, and can even relieve back pain. Enzymes tend to speed up the rate at which many bodily processes work, and injuries are no exception. Enzymes working at the site of an injury go to work to remove damaged tissue, which reduces swelling, and to help the body repair itself. As the enzymes do their work, they also become an effective pain reliever. The enzymes trypsin, chymotrypsin, papain and bromelain have been most commonly used in the studies involving enzymes and pain relief.

THE DIGESTIVE ENZYMES—NATURE'S WONDER WORKERS

Most enzymes are extremely tiny and found in very small quantities in the body. They work in organs, blood and tissue. The digestive enzymes, however, are a different story. Although you still need a microscope to see them, they are much larger than most other enzymes, and are present in the digestive system in large amounts. Since each digestive enzyme works with a specific food, a shortage or absence of even a single enzyme can make all the difference between health and sickness.

Enzymes are the catalysts in the digestive process. Food only becomes useful to the body after it has been converted to its component carbohydrates, proteins and fats in the digestive process. Only after digestion can valuable vitamins, minerals and amino acids be released and absorbed to keep us alive and healthy. The digestive enzymes cause biological reactions in our digestive systems without themselves being changed.

Each digestive enzyme works on a specific food type to break it down for absorption. One enzyme cannot substitute for another or do another's work. Enzymes that end in -ase are named by the food substance they act upon. For example, the enzyme that acts on phosphorus is named phosphatase; one of the enzymes that works on sugar (sucrose) is called sucrase.

As nutrients move through the digestive system and into the cells, they are helped along in the process by at least one enzyme. Although an enzyme is a protein, in order for it to work properly, it needs an amino acid and a coenzyme. Most coenzymes are vitamins and minerals. Two of the most important mineral coenzymes are magnesium and zinc. Magnesium alone is an essential co-factor (meaning it won't work without the magnesium present) for more than 300 different enzymes. Other minerals include iron, copper, manganese, selenium and molybdenum. The B vitamins thiamin, riboflavin, pantothenic acid and biotin are all coenzymes that help us digest starches, fats and proteins.

There are four known categories of digestive or hydrolytic enzymes:

1. **Amylase** or **amylolytic enzymes** are found in the saliva, pancreas, and intestines. They aid in the breakdown of carbohydrates.

2. **Protease** or **proteolytic enzymes** are found in the stomach, pancreas and intestines. They aid in the breakdown of proteins.

3. **Lipase** or **lipolytic enzymes** aid in the breakdown of fats.

4. **Cellulase** aids in breaking down cellulose.

AMYLASE ENZYMES THAT DIGEST STARCHES

Alpha-amylase is found in saliva and in the pancreas. It helps break down starches into sugars.

Beta-amylase is found in raw, unprocessed grains and vegetables, and also helps break down starch to sugar.

Mylase and **glucomylase** are starch-digesting enzymes capable of dissolving thousands of times their own weight in starches in the small intestine.

PROTEASE ENZYMES THAT DIGEST PROTEINS

Prolase is a concentrated protein-digesting enzyme derived from papain, which is extracted from papaya.

Protease is also extracted from papaya.

Bromelain is a digestive enzyme derived from pineapple.

Pepsin is released in the stomach, and splits protein into amino acids. In supplements, pepsin is made from animal enzymes.

Trypsin and **chymotrypsin,** produced by the pancreas, break down proteins.

Renin causes milk to coagulate, changing its protein, casein, into a form the body can use. Renin also releases minerals from milk, such as calcium, phosphorus, potassium and iron.

Pancreatin is an enzyme derived from the sections of an animal pancreas. This enzyme functions best in the small intestine.

HOW LIPASE WORKS

The efficient breakdown of fats plays a critical role in our health. Lipase and phospholipase act to break down fats in many stages, beginning with the upper portion of the stomach, called the cardial region. Here the lipase enzymes work in the acidic environment of the stomach to produce specific breakdown substances. If we aren't supplying enough enzymes here and in the main portion of the stomach to break down the fat we eat, when it reaches the small intestines it puts a much bigger load on the pancreas. The lipases supplied by the pancreas only work in the alkalinity of the small intestines, producing a whole different set of fat breakdown products than the acidic environment of the stomach. An enzyme supplement can greatly aid the digestive system by making sure that fats we eat are well down the road to digestion by the time they reach the small intestine.

HOW TO TAKE DIGESTIVE ENZYMES

When you take a digestive enzyme, be sure to take one that includes the three major types of enzymes: amylase, protease (or proteolytic enzymes) and lipase. If you eat dairy products and want some help digesting the lactose in them, get an enzyme supplement that contains lactase. Take them just before or with meals.

CHAPTER 7

How Drugs Can Deplete Nutrients

In North America we are addicted to drugs, and I don't mean the street drugs. It would probably be more accurate to say that our doctors and our mainstream medical system are addicted to drugs. The medical mind set is to diagnose a disease and then prescribe a pill for it. Very little thought is given to what caused the disease in the first place, or whether lifestyle changes and nutrition could correct the disease. As a result, Americans, and particularly older Americans, are, on the average, taking from three to eight drugs.

I call this the drug treadmill. You go to get a physical checkup with your doctor after the age of 50, and if you have slightly high cholesterol or blood pressure, if your joints hurt, or if your blood sugar is a bit off balance, you're likely to be put on a drug, with no suggestion that dietary changes or exercise might help. That drug will cause side effects. When you complain of these side effects to your doctor, you will be prescribed another drug, which in turn will cause a new set of side effects, for which you will be prescribed yet another drug, and so on. Pretty soon you're feeling tired all the time, you're depressed, gaining weight, can't sleep, have a chronic cough and no sex drive. You're not exercising any more and you're drinking twice as much coffee and eating twice as much sugar to try to bring your energy up. If you complain to your doctor about all the drugs and all the side effects, you will be threatened with the dire consequences of going off the drugs and told the side effects are simply part of old age. Hogwash!

First, I want you to know that nearly all the diseases of old age can be very well managed naturally with herbs and supplements that have few or no side effects. And most of these ailments can be prevented or reversed simply by lifestyle changes that include drinking plenty of fresh, clean water, getting some moderate exercise, cutting down on fat (particularly the hydrogenated oils) and sugar, eating plenty of fresh vegetables and taking some supplements. There is no reason why the vast majority of us can't enjoy a relatively pain-free old age with energy and vigor.

Nearly all the prescription and over-the-counter drugs prescribed by your doctor will have side effects. In the following pages I am going to list some nutrients that are depleted by some of the more common drugs. But I want you to educate yourself. There are many books available now on prescription drugs that can be understood by the average person. Read up on the drugs you're taking to find out if they are really safe and effective and what the side effects are. And even more important, take the steps to get off the drugs (with your doctor's guidance please) and take care of yourself.

Many prescription drugs cause depletion of the body's essential vitamins and minerals. A recent scientific study shows that ingredients found in common over-the-counter (OTC) cold, pain and allergy remedies actually lower the blood level of vitamin A in animals. Because vitamin A protects and strengthens the mucous membranes lining the nose, throat and lungs, a deficiency of vitamin A could actually break down these membranes, giving bacteria a cozy home to multiply in. Therefore, the drugs that are supposed to alleviate the cold may be actually prolonging it!

ASPIRIN

Aspirin is being touted as the new wonder drug to take for everything from heart disease to colon cancer. These claims are very flimsy and based more on advertising than on reality. You should know that 4,000 people die from the side effects of aspirin every year, and an additional 60,000 are hospitalized. Aspirin is well-known for causing gastrointestinal bleeding, and even a small amount of aspirin can *triple* the excretion rate of vitamin C from the body. In addition, aspirin can contribute to a deficiency of folic acid, one of the B vitamins. A deficiency of folic acid can lead to anemia, digestive disturbances, graying hair and growth problems. Taking aspirin at night will reduce the production of the hormone melatonin, and may result in insomnia.

CORTICOSTEROIDS

In spite of their horrendous side effects if used long-term, including bone loss and fragile skin, millions of people are dependent on corticosteroids such as Prednisone. These belong to a class of drugs called cortisones, used to ease the pain of arthritis, relieve lung congestion, and treat autoimmune diseases. They are also prescribed for skin problems and blood and eye disorders. Researchers conducted a study of 24 asthmatics using cortisone-type drugs and found the zinc levels were 42 percent lower than in patients not treated with corticosteroids. A zinc deficiency can lead to loss of taste and smell as well as a loss in sexual desire. Zinc is necessary for male potency and the health of the prostate gland. Zinc also enhances wound healing and is essential for a clear complexion.

BIRTH CONTROL PILLS

Oral contraceptives are made from a synthetic hormone that can lead to a deficiency of zinc, folic acid, vitamins C, B_6 and B_{12}. Deficiency of B_{12} can lead to emotional mood swings. B_6 deficiency can cause depression (many women on the pill are depressed). Women taking oral contraceptives (birth control pills) should take at least an extra 25-50 mg of B_6, 1,000 mcg of B_{12}, 400 mg of folic acid and 1,000 mg of vitamin C. Low vitamin C levels may account for increased susceptibility to blood clotting. I would recommend that you use another method of birth control, as the Pill raises your risk of strokes and cancer and causes many unpleasant side effects.

ANTACIDS

Antacids are routinely prescribed for digestive complaints such as heartburn or ulcers. In truth, what most people need is to cut back on the coffee, sugar, fatty, greasy and spicy foods, eat less, and to exercise more. Antacids interfere with the proper absorption of nutrients. Antacids that contain aluminum disturb calcium and phosphorus metabolism. Phosphorus deficiency, which is very rare (except in antacid users), can cause fatigue, loss of appetite and fragile bones.

DIURETICS

Diuretics, which are commonly prescribed for high blood pressure, also flush potassium and other minerals out of the body. Even potassium-sparing diuretics do not spare other minerals. You should be doubling your intake of minerals if you're taking diuretics.

PART II
Putting Together Your
Personal Vitamin Plan

CHAPTER 8

My Basic Adult
Vitamin-Mineral Program

Not everyone requires the same vitamins/minerals. But
here is my basic program, which you can then adapt
according to the guidelines in the following pages for
specific ages and problems. There are many multiple
vitamins available that will give you the dosages listed
below. Look for one that dissolves easily, is small enough
to swallow easily, that uses natural not synthetic vitamins,
and that doesn't use binders, fillers or colorings.

Ideally you'll take a high-potency multiple vitamin
at least twice a day that gives you:

Beta-carotene or carotenoids, 10,000-15,000 IU

The B vitamins, including:
    B_1 (thiamine), 25-50 mg
    B_2 (riboflavin), 25-100 mg
    B_3 (niacin), 25-100 mg
    B_5 (pantothenic acid), 25-100 mg
    B_6 (pyridoxine), 50-100 mg
    B_{12} (cobalamin) 100-1,000 mcg
    Biotin, 100-300 mcg
    Choline, 25-100 mg
    Folic acid, 200-400 mcg
    Inositol, 100-300 mg

Vitamin D, 100-500 IU

Vitamin C, 1000-3000 mg

Vitamin E, at least 400 IU

Minerals
Boron, 1-5 mg
Calcium (citrate, lactate or gluconate), 100-500 mg
(women should take a total of 600-1,200 mg daily)
Chromium (picolinate), 200-400 mcg
Copper, 1-5 mg
Magnesium (citrate or gluconate), 100-500 mg (women
should take a total of 300-600 mg daily)
Manganese (citrate or chelate), 10 mg
Selenium, 25-50 mcg
Vanadium (vanadyl sulfate), 25-200 mcg
Zinc, 10-15 mg

Since vitamin C, vitamin E, calcium and magnesium
tend to make a multivitamin pill larger, you can take
a multivitamin with smaller amounts of those vitamins
and then take the others separately. A calcium/mag-
nesium combination works well at bedtime when it
will help you relax and prevent leg cramps.

CHAPTER 9

Vitamins for Children

Children's nutritional needs are different from adults not only because they're growing, but also because they're smaller.

Your doctor can recommend liquid vitamins for infants and toddlers. If you are vegetarian, I recommend an additional amino acid supplement that includes all of the essential amino acids plus histidine, taurine and cysteine, which are essential for growing children.

Here are recommendations for children from the age of four to pre-puberty, around the age of 11-13.

Vitamin A/beta-carotene   500-1,000 IU

The B vitamins, including:
   B_1 (thiamine), .9-1.3 mg
   B_2 (riboflavin), 1.1-1.5 mg
   B_3 (niacin), 12-17 mg
   B_5 (pantothenic acid), 4-50 mg
   B_6 (pyridoxine), 1.1-2 mg
   B_{12} (cobalamin), 3-5 mcg
   Biotin, 50-150 mcg
   Folic acid, 150-350 mcg

Vitamin D, 100 IU

Vitamin C, 150-500 mg

Vitamin E, 15-25 IU

Minerals

Calcium (citrate, lactate or gluconate), 800 mg

Chromium (picolinate), 80-200 mcg

Iron, 10-12 mg

Magnesium (citrate or gluconate), 200-300 mg

Selenium, 100-200 mcg

Zinc, 10 mg

Bioflavonoids (amount varies with the type, but they will enhance the action of the rest of the vitamins)

CHAPTER 10

Vitamins for Teens

Minimizing the consumption of junk food, maximizing the consumption of vegetables, and daily aerobic exercise is the best health program a teen can follow. Plenty of clean water will play a major role in preventing acne and clearing the body of toxins.

CALCIUM AND BONES

Please be sure they are getting enough calcium, as good bone growth in the teens can prevent osteoporosis later in life. A diet with too much protein (more than 2 ounces per day), and too many sodas containing phosphorus will leach calcium from the bones and can be the cause of osteoporosis later in life. Milk is not a very good source of calcium, because it has a poor calcium to magnesium ratio, and the bone building doesn't happen without magnesium. If your teens are milk drinkers, please have them take a magnesium tablet with their milk. Fresh vegetables are a much better source of calcium. Exercise is also one of the best ways to build strong bones, and will help balance the surges of hormones teens have to cope with.

ACNE

If your teens are having problems with acne, you can add a vitamin A supplement, 5,000 IU, an additional 400 IU of vitamin E, and a B-complex vitamin until it clears up. Avoiding refined carbohydrates such as cakes and cookies and fried foods will help tremendously. Yogurt is the best acne-prevention food a teen can eat, and will also supply calcium. Buy plain yogurt and sweeten it with fruit.

DEPRESSION

If your teen is suffering from depression, try a B-complex vitamin and some exercise.

BASIC RECOMMENDATIONS

Vitamin A/beta-carotene   5,000 IU

The B vitamins, including:
B_1 (thiamine), 1.5 mg
B_2 (riboflavin), 2 mg
B_3 (niacin), 18 mg
B_5 (pantothenic acid), 50 mg
B_6 (pyridoxine), 2.5 mg
B_{12} (cobalamin), 5 mcg
Biotin, 75-150 mcg
Folic acid, 200 mcg

Vitamin D, 100 IU

Vitamin C, 300-500 mg

Vitamin E, 50-100 IU

Minerals
Calcium (citrate, lactate or gluconate), 1,200 mg
Chromium (picolinate), 200 mcg
Iron, 18 mg
Magnesium (citrate or gluconate), 350-400 mg
Selenium, 200 mcg
Zinc, 10-15 mg

CHAPTER 11

Vitamins for Athletes

Athletes have special vitamin needs, as their metabolism tends to be higher than average, creating a greater need for some vitamins. In addition, exercise creates free radicals, so extra protection is needed. Please be sure to drink at least 8-10 glasses of clean water every day.

Here are some guidelines for athletes:

ANTIOXIDANT PROTECTION

Take an extra antioxidant supplement containing vitamin C, vitamin E, beta carotene, selenium, and a bioflavonoid antioxidant such as green tea extract, PCO's (grapeseed extract), rutin, hesperidin, quercetin, or a combination.

OPTIMAL HEALING

To speed healing of tissue and tendon injuries, in addition to the Basic Program for Adults, take:

Vitamin C 1,000 to 3,000 mg in divided doses, daily
Calcium pantothenate (vitamin B_5), 100 mg, 1-2 times daily
Vitamin B complex, 50 mg, twice daily
Vitamin D, 400 IU daily
Glucosamine sulfate (follow instructions on the bottle)
Ginkgo biloba

WEIGHT REDUCTION

Athletes who are trying to reduce their weight can take the following nutrients to enhance fat burning:

Chromium picolinate, 200 mcg daily
Carnitine (L-carnitine or N-acetyl carnitine), 500 mg once daily
Phenylalanine, 200-500 mg daily, ½ between meals, with water (Not to be used by anyone with PKU, skin cancer or high blood pressure. If you get headaches or dizziness, stop taking it.)

WEIGHT GAIN

The best key to weight gain is to shun the sugar and junk food and go for nutrition-packed foods such as avocados, nuts and seeds, sweet potatoes, dates, raisins and moderate amounts of cheese.

Vitamins that can improve appetite include:
Vitamin B-complex, 50 mg
Vitamin B_{12}, sublingual or intranasal

CHAPTER 12

Vitamins for Women

Women can have special vitamin needs depending on age and hormone balance.

PMS

There is no single solution or easy answer to premenstrual syndrome (PMS), because each woman who suffers from it may have a variety of symptoms and causes. However, there are a few things women can try that help nearly all women with PMS to some extent.

The first thing to try is a healthy diet and exercise: cut way back on refined sugars and carbohydrates, eliminate fried foods, emphasize whole grains and fresh vegetables, eat plenty of legumes, including soy products, and drink plenty of clean water.

If that doesn't work, try the supplements listed below, and if that doesn't work, try some natural progesterone cream. (See "Osteoporosis" below for details on natural progesterone).

In addition to the Basic Adult Program, daily vitamins for PMS include the following. They can either be taken premenstrually or throughout the month.

Vitamin B$_6$, 100-300 mg daily
Beta-carotene, 15,000 to 20,000 IU daily in divided doses
Choline, 500 mg
Inositol, 500 mg

Vitamin C, 1,000 mg
Vitamin E, 400 IU
Magnesium, 300 mg

PREMENOPAUSE

Many women today are suffering from "premenopause syndrome," caused by anovulatory (not ovulat-
ing) menstrual cycles in which no progesterone is
made, creating a relative excess of estrogen. The symptoms of premenopause syndrome include weight gain,
bloating, mood swings, cold hands and feet, irritability, unstable blood sugar, fatigue, and depression. The
treatment is the same as for PMS, and may require
extra support to the adrenal glands. For a detailed
explanation of premenopause syndrome and other
women's hormone balance issues, I highly recommend the book *What Your Doctor May Not Tell You About
Menopause: The Breakthrough Book on Natural Progesterone,* by John R. Lee, M.D. (Warner Books, 1996).

OSTEOPOROSIS

It is especially important that all women get enough
calcium to prevent osteoporosis, preferably through
fresh vegetables, especially the leafy green ones.
Women who drink a lot of phosphorus-containing
sodas and eat too much protein (more than 1.5
ounces per day) will lose calcium from their bones
regardless of how much calcium they take. Please eat
a plant-based diet with plenty of soy foods and strictly
limit your intake of sodas. It is also important to get
weight-bearing exercise, which builds bone.

I also recommend that all menopausal women at
risk for osteoporosis use a natural progesterone
cream, which actually stimulates bone building and
can reverse osteoporosis as well as prevent it. Estrogen

(such as Premarin) only slows bone loss for a few years around the time of menopause and creates a high risk of cancer, so for most women I don't recommend it. Natural progesterone has no known side effects and may actually be protective against breast cancer.

By "natural progesterone cream" I don't mean the synthetic progestins such as Provera, nor do I mean the "wild yam extract" creams containing diosgenin, a laboratory precursor of progesterone. To confuse matters even further, both the creams containing natural progesterone and those containing diosgenin may be labeled "wild yam extract." Your best bet is to use a reputable source. I recommend that to find out more about how to order and use natural progesterone cream, call Professional Technical Services in Eugene, Oregon at 1-800-888-6814.

Women at risk for osteoporosis should take the following supplements, in addition to the Basic Adult Program:

Vitamin B$_6$, 50 mg/day
Calcium/magnesium, 600 mg calcium/300 mg magnesium

MENOPAUSE

Menopausal women are at higher risk of heart disease and osteoporosis, but I promise you, estrogen is not the solution! After an initial period of feeling better, estrogen and the synthetic progestins cause most women to feel as if they have permanent PMS! The not-found-in-nature synthetic hormones prescribed by most doctors do vastly more harm than good, and their ability to protect against heart disease and osteoporosis is grossly exaggerated by pharmaceutical companies eager to cash in on the discomfort of millions of menopausal women.

The problems associated with menopause are also grossly exaggerated by the drug companies and the media. In truth, it is women who have had a hysterectomy (instant menopause) who have the most problems. The vast majority of other women pass through menopause relatively uneventfully.

Your best bet for preventing and relieving menopause symptoms such as hot flashes and vaginal dryness is plenty of exercise, clean water and a nutrition-rich, low-fat diet emphasizing vegetables and soy products. Menopause symptoms are virtually nonexistent in Japan, where fat consumption is low and soy consumption is high.

Any woman with the menopause symptoms listed above and/or hair loss, dry skin, and decreased libido not relieved by the above lifestyle guidelines plus the vitamins below, should try natural progesterone cream. (See the section on osteoporosis for more information on natural progesterone.) Any woman at risk for heart disease or osteoporosis should also be using natural progesterone cream. Recent research indicates that natural progesterone may also be protective against breast cancer.

In addition to the Basic Adult Program, vitamins for women with menopause symptoms should include:

Vitamin B_6, 100-300 mg daily
Beta-carotene, 15,000 to 20,000 IU daily in divided doses
Choline, 500 mg
Inositol, 500 mg
Vitamin C, 1,000 mg
Vitamin E, 400 IU
Magnesium, 300 mg

CHAPTER 13

Vitamins for Pregnant Women

Pregnant women have special vitamin needs both to support the growing fetus and to support themselves. There are also supplements to avoid when you are pregnant. The best rule of thumb when considering whether to take any type of supplement, pill or potion when pregnant is: when in doubt, don't.

And remember, no vitamin regimen is a substitute for a balanced diet of wholesome foods including whole grains, fresh fruits and vegetables, legumes, and moderate amounts of protein.

The Basic Adult Program will work well with pregnancy, with the following changes and cautions:

Folic acid is an extremely important vitamin in preventing birth defects such as neural tube defects (spina bifida). Women of child-bearing age who are at any risk of getting pregnant should be taking 400 mcg of folic acid daily.

Women experiencing morning sickness can take 30-50 mg of vitamin B_6, which should solve the problem.

If you are suffering from varicose veins or other signs of poor circulation in the extremities, you can take the recommended dose of a standardized ginkgo biloba extract.

Vitamins women should avoid during pregnancy include vitamin A (use beta carotene), and please don't overdo it on the iron—no more than 30 mg daily.

Pregnant women should take extra calcium and magnesium, 600 mg of calcium and 300 mg of magnesium, and extra zinc for a total of 25 mg. The calcium and magnesium should be taken separately from the iron, because they can interfere with iron absorption.

The problem of preeclampsia, also called toxemia, or pregnancy-induced high blood pressure, is nearly always caused by a magnesium deficiency. Your best bet is to prevent it by taking magnesium from day one.

A pregnancy multiple vitamin should contain all the essential minerals and the trace minerals chromium, manganese and molybdenum.

Vitamins for Men

Men have special vitamin needs, mostly based on the fact of aging and declining hormone production. Men with an active sex life can also deplete vitamins E, selenium and zinc which are found in high concentrations in semen.

STRESS VITAMINS

Men who are under stress should take the following supplements daily, in addition to the Basic Adult Program:

Zinc, 15 mg
Selenium, 100 mcg
Vitamin B complex, 50 mg
Vitamin A, 5,000 IU
Vitamin C, 1,000 mg
Vitamin E, 400 IU

PROSTATE PROBLEMS

Men who have an enlarged prostate or are having symptoms of an enlarged prostate such as getting up repeatedly during the night to urinate, dribbling, and urgency, should take the following supplements in addition to the Basic Adult Program:

Zinc, 15 mg
Selenium, 100 mcg

Vitamin E, 400 IU
Vitamin B complex, 50 mg
Saw palmetto berries and pygeum extract (follow
    directions on the bottle)
Pumpkin seeds, eat a handful daily (unsalted, raw)

INCREASED SEX DRIVE

Supplements that can improve libido include:

Tyrosine, 250-500 mg daily
Phenylalanine, 250-500 mg daily
Vitamin A, 5,000 to 10,000 IU daily
Vitamin C, 1,000 mg daily
Siberian ginseng in tea, capsules or tincture
Lecithin (granules or capsules), be sure it's fresh
    and not rancid

Vitamins for Seniors

As we age we have special vitamin needs for a variety of reasons. One is that the signals from the hypothalamus and pituitary glands that regulate hormones wane, and the other is that digestion and absorption of nutrients become less efficient, vastly decreasing the amount of nutrients taken in by the body, even with a good diet. This makes supplements especially important as part of an antiaging program.

Over and over again, studies have shown that eating plenty of fresh vegetables and moderate exercise are two of your keys to a healthy and energetic old age.

For more detail on the foods, herbs and supplements that work to slow the aging process, I recommend my books, *Earl Mindell's Anti-Aging Bible* (Simon & Schuster, 1996) and *Dr. Earl Mindell's What You Should Know about the Super Antioxidant Miracle* (Keats Publishing, 1996).

Here are the extra supplements I recommend for seniors in addition to the Basic Adult Program:

Glucosamine sulfate (for stiff joints), follow directions on bottle

Betaine hydrochloride (to aid digestion), follow directions on bottle

Digestive enzymes (follow directions on bottle)

Vitamin B_{12}, 1,000 mg every three days, sublingually or intranasally

Vitamin B_6, 50 mg daily

Folic acid, 100 mcg daily

Bioflavonoid antioxidant formula (for example, rutin, hesperidin, PCO's as grapeseed extract, green tea extract, quercetin)

Ginkgo biloba (follow directions on the bottle)

Melatonin (if you're having trouble sleeping), 1.5 mg 1 hour before bed

Magnesium, 300 mg daily

Glutathione (take N-acetyl cysteine, a precursor), follow directions on bottle

Coenzyme Q10, 30-90 mg daily

L-carnitine, 500-1,000 mg daily

Ginseng (when recovering from illness or for stamina)

GLOSSARY

absorption The process by which nutrients are passed into the bloodstream.

acetate A derivative of **acetic acid.**

acetic acid Used as a synthetic flavoring agent, one of the first food additives (vinegar is approximately 4 to 6 per cent acetic acid); it is found naturally in cheese, coffee, grapes, peaches, raspberries and strawberries. Generally Recognized As Safe **(GRAS)** when used only in packaging.

acetylcholine One of the chemicals involved in the transmission of nerve impulses.

adrenalin(e) A hormone secreted by the **adrenal glands** into the bloodstream in response to physical or mental stress, such as fear or injury; works with **noradrenalin(e)** to regulate blood pressure and heart rate.

adrenal glands The glands, located above each kidney, that manufacture **adrenalin(e), noradrenalin(e),** and **steroids.**

aldosterone A hormone secreted by the **adrenal glands** which regulates the salt and water balance in the body; one of the **steroids.**

alkaline Containing an acid-neutralizing substance (being alkaline, sodium bicarbonate is used for excess acidity in foods).

allergen A substance that causes an **allergy.**

159

amino acid chelates Chelated minerals that have been produced by many of the same processes nature uses to **chelate** minerals in the body; in the digestive tract, nature surrounds the elemental minerals with **amino acid,** permitting them to be absorbed into the bloodstream.

amino acids The organic compounds from which proteins are constructed; 22 amino acids have been identified as necessary to the human body; 9 are known as essential—histidine, isoleucine, leucine, lysine, total S-containing amino acids, total aromatic amino acids, threonine, tryptophan, and valine—and must be obtained from food.

amenorrhea Absence or suppression of menstruation.

androgen Any of the group of hormones which stimulates male characteristics.

angina pectoris A cramping pain in the chest, stemming from the heart and often spreading to the left shoulder and arm.

anorexia Loss of appetite, especially resulting from disease.

anorexia nervosa A psychophysiological disorder featuring an abnormal fear of becoming obese, a persistent aversion to food, a distorted self-image, and severe loss of weight.

antibody A protein substance produced in the blood or tissues in response to a specific **antigen,** such as a **toxin** or bacteria; by neutralizing **organic** poisons and weakening or destroying bacteria, antibodies form the basis of immunity.

antigen Any substance not normally present in the body that stimulates the body to produce antibodies.

antihistamine A drug used to reduce effects associated with **histamine** production in allergies and colds.

antineoplastics Drugs that prevent the growth and development of malignant cells.

antioxidant A substance that can protect another substance from **oxidation**; added to foods to keep oxygen from changing the food's color.

antitoxin An **antibody** formed in response to, and capable of neutralizing, a poison of biological origin.

arthritis Inflammation of joints.

arteriosclerosis A disease of the arteries characterized by hardening, thickening, and loss of elasticity of the arterial walls; results in impaired blood circulation.

assimilation The process whereby nutrients are used by the body and changed into living tissue.

asthma A condition of lungs characterized by a decrease in diameter of some air passages; a spasm of the bronchial tubes or swelling of their mucous membranes.

ataxia Loss of coordinated movement caused by disease of the nervous system.

atherosclerosis A process where fatty deposits in the walls of arteries make the walls thick and hard, narrowing the arteries; a form of **arteriosclerosis**.

ATP A molecule called adenosine triphosphate, the fuel of life, a nucleotide—building block of **nucleic acid**—that produces biological energy with vitamins B_1, B_2, B_3, and pantothenic acid, another B complex **vitamin**.

autoimmunity An abnormal condition where the body produces antibodies against its own tissues.

avidin A protein in egg white capable of inactivating **biotin**.

bacteriophage A **virus** that infects bacteria.

basal metabolic rate The body's rate of metabolism when at rest.

basophil A type of white blood cell representing less than 1% of the total.

B cells White blood cells, made in bone marrow, which produce antibodies upon instructions from T cells, manufactured in the **thymus**.

beta-carotene A plant pigment which can be converted into two forms of **vitamin A**.

BHA Butylated hydroxyanisole; a preservative and **antioxidant** used in many products; insoluble in water; can be toxic to the kidneys.

BHT Butylated hydroxytoluene; a solid, white crystalline **antioxidant** used to retard spoilage of many foods; can be more toxic to the kidney than its nearly identical chemical cousin, **BHA**.

bioflavonoids A group of compounds needed to maintain healthy blood vessel walls; found chiefly as coloring matter in flowers and fruits, particularly yellow ones; known as vitamin P complex.

biotin A colorless, crystalline B complex **vitamin**; essential for the activity of many **enzyme** systems; helps produce **fatty acids**; found in large quantities in liver, egg yolk, milk, and yeast.

bursa A pouch or sac containing fluid for the lubrication of joints.

bursitis Swelling or inflammation of a **bursa**.

calciferol A colorless, odorless crystalline material, insoluble in water; soluble in fats; a synthetic form of **vitamin** D made by irradiating **ergosterol** with ultraviolet light.

calcium gluconate An **organic** calcium based compound.

capillary A minute blood vessel, one of many that connect the arteries and veins and deliver oxygen to tissues.

carcinogen A cancer-causing substance.

cardiotonic A compound which aids the heart.

cardiovascular Relating to the heart and blood vessels.

carotene An orange-yellow pigment occuring in many plants and capable of being converted into **vitamin** A in the body.

casein The **protein** in milk that has become the standard by which protein quality is measured.

catabolism The metabolic change of nutrients or complex substances into simpler compounds, accompanied by a release of energy.

catalyst A substance that modifies, especially increases, the rate of chemical reaction without being consumed or changed in the process.

cellulose Carbohydrate found in the outer layers of fruits and vegetables which is undigestible.

cerebrovascular accident A blood clot or bleeding in the brain; a stroke.

chelation A process by which mineral substances are changed into an easily digestible form.

cholesterol A white, crystalline substance, made up of various fats; naturally produced in vertebrate animals and humans; important as a precursor to steroid hormones and as a constituent of cell membranes.

chronic Of long duration, continuing, constant.

CNS Central nervous system.

coenzyme A substance that combines with other substances to form a complete **enzyme**; nonprotein and usually a B **vitamin**.

collagen The primary **organic** constituent of bone, cartilage and connective tissue (becomes gelatin through boiling).

complex carbohydrate Fibrous molecules of starch or sugar which slowly release sugar into the bloodstream.

congenital Condition existing at birth, not hereditary.

coronary occlusion Blockage of a heart artery.

coronary thrombosis Blood clot in a heart artery.

corticosteroids See **steroids.**

dermatitis An inflammation of the skin; a rash.

diastolic Second number in a blood pressure reading; measures the pressure in arteries between contractions of the heart.

dicalcium phosphate A filler used in pills, which is derived from purified mineral rocks and is a source of calcium and phosphorus.

demineralization The loss of minerals or salts from bone and tissue.

diluents Fillers; inert material added to tablets to increase their bulk in order to make them a practical size for compression.

disaccharide A sugar which breaks down into two **monosaccharides.**

diuretic Tending to increase the flow of urine from the body.

DNA Deoxyribonucleic acid; the **nucleic acid** in chromosomes that is part of the chemical basis for hereditary characteristics.

emulsion A substance with chemical characteristics of both water and oil; aids mixing and dispersing between the two.

endocrine Producing secretions passed directly to the **lymph** or blood instead of into a duct; to do with the endocrine glands or the **hormones** they produce.

endogenous Being produced from within the body.

endorphins Natural opiates produced in the brain; pain suppressants.

enteric coated A tablet coated so that it dissolves in the intestine, not in the acid environment of the stomach.

enzyme A **protein** substance found in living cells that brings about chemical changes; necessary for digestion of food; compounds with names ending in -*ase*.

epinephrine See **adrenalin(e)**

ergosterol A **vitamin** D group **steroid**; originally found in ergot, a fungal disease of rye; also found in other fungi, yeast, and mushrooms; changed by ultraviolet light into vitamin D_2

excipient Any inert substance used as a dilutant or vehicle for a drug.

exogenous Being derived or developed from external causes.

fatty acid Acids produced by the breakdown of fats; essential fatty acids cannot be produced by the body and must be included in the diet.

FDA Food and Drug Administration.

fibrin An insoluble **protein** that forms the necessary fibrous network in the coagulation of blood. An excess of fibrinogen in the blood increases the risk of heart disease.

free radicals Highly reactive chemical fragments that can beneficially act as chemical messengers, but in excess produce an irritation of artery walls and start the arteriosclerotic process if antioxidants are not present.

fructose A natural sugar occurring in fruits and honey, called fruit sugar; often used as a preservative for foodstuffs and an intravenous nutrient.

galactosemia A hereditary disorder in which ingested milk becomes toxic.

gland An organ in the body where certain substances in the blood are seperated and converted into secretions for use in the body (such as hormones) or to be discharged from the body (such as sweat); nonsecreting structures similar to glands, like **lymph** nodes, are also known as glands.

glucose Blood sugar; a product of the body's **assimilation** of carbohydrates and a major source of energy.

glutamic acid An **amino acid** present in all complete proteins; also manufactured commercially from vegetable protein; used as a salt substitute and a flavor-intensifying agent.

glutamine An **amino acid** that constitutes, with **glucose**, the major nourishment used by the nervous system.

gluten A mixture of two proteins, gliadin and glutenin, present in wheat, rye, oats, and barley.

glycogen The body's chief form of stored carbohydrate, primarily in the liver; coverted to **glucose** when needed.

GRAS Generally Recognized as Safe; a list established by Congress to cover substances added to food.

HDL High-density lipoprotein; HDL is sometimes called "good" **cholesterol** because it is the body's major carrier of cholesterol to the liver for excretion in the bile.

hemoglobin Molecule necessary for the transport of oxygen by red blood cells; iron is an essential component.

hesperidin Part of the **vitamin** C complex.

histamine An **organic** compound of ammonia released by the body in allergic reactions.

holistic treatment Treatment of the whole person, rather than just parts or symptoms.

homeostasis The body's physiological equilibrium.

hormone A substance formed in **endocrine** organs and transported by body fluids to activate other specifically receptive organs, cells or tissues.

humectant A substance that is used to preserve the moisture content of materials.

hydrochloric acid An acid secreted in the stomach; a main part of gastric juice.

hydrolyzed Put into water-soluble form.

hydrolyzed protein chelate Water-soluble and chelated for easy **assimilation.**

hyperglycemia A condition caused by high blood sugar.

hypoglycemia A condition caused by abnormally low blood sugar.

ichthyosis A condition characterized by a scaliness on the outer layer of skin.

idiopathic A condition whose causes are not yet known.

immune Protected against disease.

infarction Localized tissue death due to lack of oxygen supply.

insulin A **hormone**, secreted by the pancreas, that helps regulate the **metabolism** of sugar in the body.

interferon Any of a group of proteins produced by cells in response to infection by a **virus**; prevents viral replication and can induce resistance to viral antigens.

IU International Units

lactose One of the sugars found in milk.

lactating Producing milk.

LDL Low-density lipoprotein; sometimes referred to as "bad" **cholesterol,** LDLs easily become **oxidized** and carry cholesterol through the bloodstream; studies show high levels can increase risk of coronary artery disease (CAD).

lecithin Any of a group of fats rich in phosphorus; essential for transforming fats in the body; rich sources include egg yolk, soybeans and corn.

linoleic acid One of the polyunsaturated fats; an essential **fatty acid**; a constituent of **lecithin**; known as **vitamin F**; indispendable for life, and must be obtained from foods.

lipid A fat or fatty substance.

lipofuscin A group of fats, plentiful in adult cells and associated with aging.

lipotropic Preventing abnormal or excessive accumulation of fat; lipotropin is a **hormone** which stimulates the conversion of stored fat to usable, liquid form.

lymph The almost clear fluid flowing through the lymphatic vessels; lymph nourishes tissue cells and returns waste matter to the bloodstream.

lymphocyte Any of the almost colorless cells produced in lymphoid tissue, as in the **lymph** nodes, spleen, thymus, and tonsils; lymphocytes make up between 22 and 28 percent of adult human white blood cells; primarily responsible for **antibody** production, lymphocytes include **B cells** and **T cells**.

megavitamin therapy Treatment of illness with massive amounts of vitamins.

metabolism The processes of physical and chemical change where food is synthesised into living matter until it is broken down into simpler substances or waste matter; energy is produced by these processes.

monosaccharide A simple sugar with one molecular unit such as **glucose**.

mucopolysaccharide Thick gelatinous material that is found in many places in the body; it glues cells together and lubricates joints.

naturopathy The use of herbs and other methods to stimulate the body's innate defenses without using drugs.

neuropathy Symptoms caused by abnormalities in sensory or motor nerves.

neurotransmitter A chemical substance which transmits or changes nerve impulses.

nitrites Used as fixatives in cured meats; can combine with natural stomach and food chemicals to cause dangerous cancer-causing agents called nitrosamines.

noradrenalin(e) A hormone produced in the **adrenal glands** that increases blood pressure by blood vessel narrowing without affecting the heart's output; works with **epinephrine**.

norepinephrine See **noradrenalin(e)**.

nucleic acid Any of a group of complex compounds which form a major part of **DNA** and **RNA**; found in all living cells and viruses.

oncologist Specialist in tumors; cancer specialist.

organic Describes any chemical containing carbon; or any food or supplement made with animal or vegetable fertilizers; or produced without synthetic fertilizers or pesticides and free from chemical injections or additives.

orthomolecular The right molecule used for the right treatment; doctors who practice preventive medicine and use vitamin therapies are known as orthomolecular physicians.

OSHA Occupational Safety and Health Administration.

oxalates Organic chemicals found in certain foods, especially spinach, which can combine with calcium to form calcium oxalate, an insoluble chemical the body cannot use.

oxidation The way in which certain types of altered oxygen molecules cause biochemical reactions; examples are browning of apples and rancidity in oil.

PABA Para-aminobenzoic acid; a member of the **vitamin** B complex.

palmitate Water-solubilized **vitamin A**.

peroxides Free radicals formed as by-products when oxygen reacts with molecules of fat.

phytoestrogen Any of a number of compounds found in plants which occupy estrogen receptors and may help protect the body from the negative effects of excess estrogen.

PKU (phenylketonuria) A hereditary disease caused by the lack of an **enzyme** needed to convert an essential **amino acid** (phenylalanine) into a form usable by the body; can cause mental retardation unless detected early.

placebo A substance which produces no pharmacological activity; one used instead of and alongside an active substance for comparison.

polysaccharide A molecule made up of many sugar molecules joined together.

polyunsaturated fats Highly nonsaturated fats from vegetable sources; can dissolve or absorb other substances.

precancerous lesion Tissue that is abnormal but not yet malignant.

predigested protein Protein that has been processed for fast **assimilation** and can go directly into the bloodstream.

prostaglandins Hormonelike substances that aid in regulation of the immune system.

protein A complex substance containing nitrogen which is essential to plant and animal cells; ingested proteins are changed to **amino acids** in the body.

provitamin A **vitamin** precursor; a chemical substance necessary to produce a **vitamin**.

PUFA Polyunsaturated **fatty acid.**

RDA Recommended Dietary Allowances as established by the Food and Nutrition Board, National Academy of Sciences, National Research Council.

retrovirus A class of viruses containing **RNA.**

riboflavin Vitamin B_2; part of the B vitamin complex; yellow, crystallike **coenzyme** involved in the breakdown of proteins, fats and carbohydrates; must be obtained from food.

ribonucleic acid (RNA) A constituent of all living cells and many viruses; its structure determines **protein** synthesis and genetic transmission.

rose hip A rich source of **vitamin** C; the nodule underneath the bud of a rose called a hip, in which the plant produces vitamin C.

rutin A substance often extracted from buckwheat; part of the **vitamin** C complex.

saturated fatty acids Usually solid at room temperature; higher proportions found in foods from animal sources.

sclerosis The hardening or thickening of a part of the body, such as an artery.

sequestrant A substance that absorbs some of the products of chemical reactions; it prevents changes that would affect flavor, texture, and color of food; used for water softening.

serotonin A **neurotransmitter** considered essential for sleep and concentration.

serum Any thin, watery fluid; especially the clear, sticky part of blood that remains after clotting.

simple carbohydrate Simple sugar molecules, such as **glucose**, which are rapidly absorbed by the bloodstream.

steroids Hormones produced by the **adrenal glands** that influence or control key functions of the body; formed from **cholesterol**; three major types influencing skin, muscle, fat, and **metabolism** of **glucose**, sexual functions and characteristics, and processing of minerals; used as drugs such as cortisone to suppress the immune system, reduce inflammation and to treat allergies.

syncope Brief loss of consciousness; fainting.

synergistic The way two or more substances produce an effect that neither alone could accomplish.

synthetic Produced artificially; not found in nature.

systemic Capable of spreading through the entire body.

systolic First number in a blood pressure reading; measures the pressure in arteries as the heart contracts.

T Cells White blood cells, manufactured in the **thymus**, which protect the body from bacteria, viruses, and cancer-causing agents, while controlling the production of **B cells** which produce antibodies, and unwanted production of potentially harmful **T cells**.

teratological Monstrous or abnormal formations in animals or plants.

thymus Major gland of the immune system situated behind the top of the breastbone; site of **T cell** production.

tocopherols The group of compounds (alpha, beta, delta, episilon, eta, gamma and zeta) that make **vitamin** E; obtained through vacuum distillation of edible vegetable oils.

toxicity The quality or condition of being poisonous, harmful, or destructive.

toxin An **organic** poison produced in living or dead organisms.

triglycerides Fatty substances in the blood.

unsaturated fatty acids Most often liquid at room temperature; primarily found in vegetable fats.

virus Any of a large group of minute organisms that can only reproduce in the cells of plants and animals.

vitamin Any of about fifteen natural compounds essential in small amounts as catalysts for processes in the body; most cannot be made by the body and must come from diet.

xerosis Skin condition of dryness, lacking moisture or oil; often resulting in a pattern of fine lines, scaling and itching.

yeast Single celled fungus that can cause infections in the body.

zyme A fermenting substance.

Dr. Earl Mindell's

What You Should
Know About
Trace Minerals

CHAPTER 1

The Role of Trace Minerals

Everyone has heard of the essential minerals calcium and magnesium, but relatively few know of the importance of the trace minerals, such as chromium, vanadium and selenium. Although the trace minerals comprise less than four percent of our total body weight, their presence, absence or imbalance can mean the difference between health and illness, and even between life and death.

Vitamins cannot function without trace minerals. Trace minerals also play a role in regulating hormones, enzymes, amino acids and the immune system. They are required to build and maintain the structure of the body, and to maintain proper brain function, blood sugar balance and to keep the intestines healthy and fully functioning. In other words, trace minerals are involved in every aspect of health and balance in the human body. While the body can synthesize some vitamins, it cannot manufacture a single trace mineral, and can withstand a deficiency of vitamins longer than a deficiency of minerals. In turn, vitamins play a role in the uptake and utilization of trace minerals.

Although trace mineral consumption is tiny compared to that of energy-providing foods, they perform fundamental chemical tasks in an extremely wide range of vital animal and plant functions. The quantities of minerals required are no measure of their importance in the human body. While many so-called major minerals such as calcium and magnesium are needed in milligram amounts, most trace minerals are needed in microgram amounts!

The minute amounts of trace minerals needed have meant their importance was largely undiscovered until the 20th century. Once uncovered, however, the activity of trace minerals opened a giant chest of subtle but very powerful tools for fine-tuning the body for optimal health, increasing the benefits of exercise, and even preventing cancer, heart disease and diabetes. Learn about trace minerals and you will have found a way to fine-tune your personal nutrition to maximize your health.

THE STORY OF MINERALS

The story of minerals is as old as the earth, with billions of years of participation in the very formation of life on this planet. Before animal and vegetable, there was mineral in the form of chemical elements such as iron and silicon. Primeval rains created the first oceans and washed minerals into the seas, quickening the pace of evolution in the first chapter of life.

The sciences of biochemistry, physics and geology continue to unravel the mysteries of the minerals needed for life. I found a *New York Times* story about sulfur of particular interest: According to this article, some researchers believe the asteroid collision thought to have led to the extinction of the dinosaurs resulted in wide distribution of the trace element sulfur. The asteroid was especially rich in sulfur and is thought to have vaporized, creating more than 100 billion tons of mainly sulfur dioxide in the atmosphere, increasing the availability of sulfur for the life forms that evolved after the dinosaurs.

WHAT ARE MINERALS?

To be technical, minerals are inorganic chemical elements. Inorganic means not bound to carbon. Sometimes minerals are described as inorganic when they have not been dissolved in water or transformed by plants. "Inorganic" minerals are harder for the body to absorb than those in organic form. While the chemical structure of the minerals themselves doesn't change, they may be attached to other molecules that give them different properties.

Since the origin of multicellular life minerals have been important for their ability to bond to themselves and other substances in animals and plants. In this way they help create important chemical compounds. The trace mineral cobalt is a component of vitamin B12, and iron is a part of hemoglobin. The total of about 22 dietary minerals are needed for optimal human health.

Rocks remain the original source of minerals, since living matter cannot synthesize them as it can most vitamins. Fortunately, we don't have to serve up pebbles and stones with meals! Nature has instead provided pathways for minerals, taking them from soil and water to plants and animals. Wise eating, drinking and use of supplements insures that we take in just enough dietary minerals to keep our bodies fully functional.

WHAT ARE TRACE MINERALS?

In a 150-pound body, some two to three pounds is the mineral calcium, which we need to get from what we eat. Vanadium, in contrast, would be difficult even to measure, and yet it is a trace mineral that can help reverse adult-onset diabetes in the form of the compound vanadyl sulfate.

The definition of what exactly a trace mineral is varies, but in general it is a mineral that makes up less than 0.01 percent of body weight. The major minerals, or macrominerals, each make up more than 0.01 percent of body weight. Although a few trace minerals such as zinc are needed in milligram amounts daily, most are needed in only microgram amounts. Trace minerals are sometimes called "trace elements," and those needed to maintain health are called "essential" trace minerals or elements.

The macrominerals essential to human health are calcium, phosphorus, magnesium, potassium, sodium and chloride. The trace minerals we will cover in some detail in this book, either because they are essential to optimal health or because they can play a key role in healing, are boron, chromium, cobalt, copper, fluorine, iodine, iron, lithium, manganese, molybdenum, selenium, vanadium and zinc. Trace minerals that are found in the body but which are poisonous in very small amounts when inhaled, absorbed or ingested include arsenic, aluminum, cadmium, lead, mercury, nickel and tin. Toxicity caused by these metals is largely a result of by-products of manufacturing and pollution.

The tiniest amounts of trace minerals are all that is needed to keep body functions running smoothly, but a deficiency has quite obvious effects. For example, in the absence of only a little over one millionth of an ounce of iodine, the thyroid gland enlarges.

The nutritional role of copper and iron may have been unknown in ancient times, but along with other minerals, they were believed to possess spiritual powers. Although the story of essential trace minerals and humans began hundreds of thousands of years ago, it remained mostly untold until the 20th century. In 1928 just three trace elements were recognized: Iron, which was found in the 17th century to be needed for healthy blood; iodine, shown in 1850 to prevent goiter (thyroid deficiency); and copper, found in 1928 to be needed for the absorption and utilization of iron. In the ensuing decades, other trace minerals were found to play a role in maintaining health. It wasn't until the '80s that boron and vanadium were added to the list of important trace minerals.

WHERE ARE TRACE MINERALS FOUND?

Trace minerals are washed from rocks into streams and lakes, and they are naturally found in food. Tiny mineral particles also form layers of subsoil and are absorbed by water passing by or through. Plants need minerals to function and have evolved methods for absorbing them efficiently from soil and water. In turn, animals meet most of their mineral needs by eating plants. Humans meet their minerals needs by eating both plants and animals, and drinking water. The cycle continues as man, animals and plants die, eventually returning their mineral content to the environment.

It is impossible to specify the quantities of any trace mineral likely to be found in foods. Soil conditions, time of year, weather, and environmental pollution all influence mineral levels. The way a trace mineral is chemically packaged within a food is as important as its quantity. Different mineral compounds are absorbed more or less easily during digestion. Spinach, for example, has traditionally been considered a rich source of iron. In fact, it contains iron oxalate, which makes the iron only partially available to the human body. Parsley offers a form of iron that is much easier for the body to assimilate.

Knowing which foods are typically high in a particular trace mineral is useful when it comes to planning a healthy diet. Just one Brazil nut (find an unshelled, organically grown one if possible) a day, for example, can provide a daily dose of selenium. However, it remains important to eat a variety of foods to increase the number of sources and varieties of trace minerals in the diet.

CHAPTER 2

Trace Minerals and Health

Copper, iron, manganese and zinc are trace minerals needed by all bacteria, algae, fungi and higher plants for survival. Boron is required by green plants and algae, while some also need cobalt and molybdenum. This has been true for billions of years, since the first primitive organisms in the world's oceans began to develop. As life evolved, relatively advanced chemical structures were created, with minerals as major components. One such structure was chlorophyll, the substance in plants which uses the energy of light to convert carbon dioxide and water to carbohydrates. At the center of chlorophyll is the major mineral magnesium. In this way, the same silver-white flaring metal used in flashbulbs and fireworks is crucial to any vegetable or part of a grazing animal you might eat.

The trace mineral molybdenum is used by blue-green algae and other plant life to turn nitrogen into a usable compound essential to all life. Wherever we turn, minerals are in action contributing to processes that are key to life on earth.

In humans, trace minerals are involved in protein, hormone and vitamin formation; immunity, muscle function, and nerve transmission. Zinc, for example, is used in practically every cell process. The strong, consistent structure of minerals makes them essential in the body's structures, from the calcium, phosphorus and boron in the bones to silicon, which is an important component of collagen, the principal structural component found in skin. Silicon forms long, complex molecules, suitable for parts of the body, like skin, that need to be strong and flexible. Vitamin C is another major component of collagen.

Minerals are well known for their role as catalysts, speeding up chemical reactions in the body. Catalysts help the formation or breakdown of substances to occur with less energy than the original chemicals involved would need on their own. Needing less energy, life processes such as digestion and healing can occur more quickly and efficiently. Without catalysts, many essential biological reactions would take place too slowly to sustain life. Throughout any reaction, in a very neat arrangement, catalysts themselves remain unchanged, ready for re-use. The trace mineral molybdenum, for example, activates an enzyme (another type of catalyst) which detoxifies harmful preservative compounds called sulfites.

You could say that minerals act as wheelbarrows, forklifts, gears, conveyor belts and electronic switches in the factory of the body, assisting at every step from unloading the fuel trucks and stoking and damping the boilers to switching the wiring and oiling the machinery.

The importance of all this work? Tachycardia—rapid heartbeat—can be caused by a lack of potassium; diabetes can be brought on by a shortage of chromium and zinc; anemia can be caused by a lack of iron through a deficiency of cobalt, which is also required in vitamin B12 and is needed for the absorption of iron.

Prevention of disease through adequate mineral uptake should be a natural result of our nutritional intake. The increasing pollution, intensive farming, deforestation, food refining and use of medical drugs during the 20th century, however, have depleted dietary minerals and increased our exposure to minerals that are toxic in small amounts. The need is greater than ever before to ensure an adequate mineral supply for anyone interested in maintaining good health.

THE ELECTROLYTE POWER OF MINERALS

The best minerals come shaken, not stirred! Minerals are at their most powerful in forms which conduct electricity. Electrically charged minerals are known as "ionized salts" or electrolytes. Electrolytes are produced naturally as minerals are swept up and tumbled by water rushing past rocks. Homeopathic medicines, often diluted forms of minerals, are produced by deliberately simulating this natural process through vigorous shaking. The electrical charge of electrolytes makes them valuable triggers of processes in cells. Ionized mineral particles are small enough to pass directly through cell walls, bypassing the digestive process, to be absorbed within minutes of being taken. In this way minerals can act as a charge to cells which, in turn are like batteries supplying energy to the body.

Solutions of ionized minerals are described as "crystalloid." Crystalloid solutions increase the availability of minerals to the body. Minerals also exist in more inert forms as part of "colloid" suspensions. Colloid is the term used for fairly large particles unable to dissolve but able to remain partially suspended in water. Minerals in colloidal form do not pass through animal and plant membranes as easily as electrolytes in crystalloid solutions. "The best of both worlds would be to microencapsulate ionized and colloidal minerals in soy phosphatide microspheres for optimum absorption through the transmucosal membranes of the mouth. This allows for rapid sublingual absorption and bypasses the harsh digestive system."

Soil and plants in good condition contain all the

ingredients necessary to ionize colloidal minerals, preparing them for absorption. Similarly, a healthy diet ensures a nutritionally balanced body that is adapted to absorb minerals. Hydrochloric acid softens minerals, making sure, with the help of vitamins, that they travel from the gut and into the bloodstream. Once in the bloodstream, vitamins and other substances help to ionize minerals as necessary which enables them to move into the tissues of the body where they are required.

Mineral supplements become necessary because modern farming, irrigation, pollution and water cleansing have produced food and water supplies robbed of electrolytes. Food produced using modern methods may be cheaper, but it is also a nutritional rip-off. Buy organic as much as you can and rest assured the extra dollars are harnessing valuable electrolyte power.

CHAPTER 3

How Minerals Are Depleted

Evolution has led to a system in which minerals move from soil and water to plants, animals and humans. Sustainability marks the beauty of the system as minerals return intact to soil and water through the rot and decay of organic matter. Until the industrial revolution of the 19th century, the cycle of minerals was mainly undisturbed and vegetables, meat, fish and dairy foods were reliable sources of most minerals.

Ironically, as science continues to reveal more and more about the value of minerals, they have become less and less easily available from food. The story behind this unhappy scenario is largely one of refined foods, medical drugs, chemical fertilizers, pollution and deforestation. The mineral depletion so evident in today's crop-growing soils and fast foods is reflected in the depleted state of health of people all over the world, with escalating rates of killer illnesses like cancer and heart disease.

Bringing our individual mineral intakes up to par is an important dietary action. It's also worth remembering that our own actions as consumers, workers, drivers and gardeners are influencing the mineral levels of the world we live in.

SOIL LOSS IS MINERAL LOSS

The mineral-rich result of 100 to 1,000 years of natural processes is one inch of topsoil rich in minerals and other nutrients. An unprotected layer of soil ten times this thick can disappear in the trail of a bulldozer or the puff of a violent storm. Environmentally unsound farming practices and the paving of civilization have led to a steady depletion of a precious natural resource the world over.

According to Bernard Jensen and Mark Anderson in the important book *Empty Harvest* (Avery Publishing, 1990), when pioneers first crossed North America they settled on land with topsoils 18 to 25 inches deep. Today, the figure in most states is around six inches, often less. Out of· the total measurement of soil erosion in the U.S., 90 percent occurs on farmland. Midwestern states like Wyoming and Nebraska have literally seen their soils blown away creating huge "dust bowls" where farmers once led a prosperous life. The days of the farming disasters of the Great Plains are still with us. North Dakota lost 3.5 million acres of topsoil to wind in 1988 alone. In the drought years of 1988-89, soil loss through wind and water was estimated at six billion tons per year.

The U.S. Department of Agriculture estimates that a six-inch loss of topsoil can reduce crop yields by 40 percent a year. Until topsoil is seen as a complex store of minerals and organic matter of great value, it will still be easy to abuse. Often soil has been seen only as a useful medium because it holds plants upright and can receive the water they need. The loss of essential dietary minerals has gone unnoticed. The remaining land has been forced to produce more food artificially and unsustainably. Salty, over-irrigated soils and creeping desert conditions are examples of the result—hardly conducive to good human nutrition.

KEEPING OUR SOIL MINERAL-RICH

In its natural state, quality soil is 45 percent minerals and is full of "good" bacteria. A teaspoon of good soil contains billions of living creatures. Soil is the major source of nutrients for most plants. Mineral-rich soil supports soil microbes that break down anything falling onto the soil, from dead leaves to picnic leftovers. In this way, matter is rotted down into its basic elements, including minerals, which then form part of the soil. This cycle keeps soil mineral-rich in a self-perpetuating cycle.

People often forget that bacteria are not usually disease agents, but actually perform very useful functions. Only when there are not enough bacteria to do the work required or the bacteria start to function where they are not needed does trouble begin. What prevents bacteria from devouring living plants? Plants are protected by a natural balance of fungi and bacteria. The fungi, called mycorrhiza, live along plant rootlets and secrete toxins which act against bacteria. The toxins, in a word, are antibiotics, just like the famous example produced from the *Penicillium* mold. By fending off bacteria, the mycorrhiza play an essential part in plant immunity and help create healthy crops.

When the uptake of minerals is out of balance, the result is deformity or deficiency. Mycorrhiza fungi help plants keep their mineral intake in balance. If mycorrhiza did not act as a buffer, plants would simply absorb minerals in proportion to the amounts found in soil. This would not necessarily match the plant's relative needs for each mineral. They perform this balancing action by binding needed minerals to protein, a process known as chelating. Chelation ensures that plants take in the minerals they need rather than the minerals in greatest quantity around them.

Healthy soil, then, is rich in bacteria that recycle matter into its basic elements which in turn help keep soil bacteria-rich. Plants benefit from the products of soil bacteria and don't get rotted down themselves because they are protected by fungi. Mycorrhiza fungi also protect plants from over- and underconsumption of the minerals they need. Such natural checks and balances in soil and plant life pay wonderful dividends to human beings in strong, healthy crops that can never be bettered by artificial, unnatural tinkering. And, of course, when we eat plants with the right balance of trace minerals, we're consuming the trace minerals essential for our own good health.

ARTIFICIAL FERTILIZERS AND PESTICIDES LEAD TO MINERAL LOSS

Topsoil loss is bad enough. The quality of the soil remaining is in many ways producing a slow starvation—not of calories, but of minerals. Since the industrial revolution and technological advances of the 19th and 20th centuries, farming itself has become an industry. Early scientific discoveries focused on boosting plant growth and killing agents of crop disease. Manmade fertilizers and pesticides did produce initial dramatic increases in crop yields and led to a large scale shift from traditional farming practices.

The invention of the tractor in the early 20th century distanced farmers even more from soil as the most vital resource of their work. Land began to be overworked and underfed at an unprecedented rate. It no longer seemed necessary to let fields lie fallow for a time or to dig crop remains back into the soil. Soil-rejuvenating crops known to host beneficial bacteria were no longer grown in years between crops reared for greater profit. Deficient soils unable to support livestock profitably were forced to grow crops for humans.

Soils in many areas have now become so deficient in enzymes, microbes, worms and insect life that crop remnants sit unrotted and do not become compost.

Science produced powerful chemicals in the form of

pesticides that could kill disease-producing organisms in plants. Pesticides changed the focus of farming from raising strong crops to treating sick ones or eliminating sources of sickness.

Chemical fertilizers are also part of the trend, substituting crop boosting for crop nurturing. Today, we pay the price of foods kept artificially free of disease and blemishes in mineral depletion and the risks that it brings.

Naturally caused inequalities will always exist in crops. Mineral variations are to be expected according to time of harvesting, climate and geology. However, the use of artificial fertilizers whose formulas are influenced by cost and profit rather than the actual needs of the soil in any given location has created unbalanced soil that is too high in some minerals and too low in others.

Chemical fertilizers contain relatively few minerals. This in itself leads to deficiencies in the "fertilized" plants. The chemical contents of artificial fertilizers are concentrated and acidic, typically mixtures of ammonia and nitrogen, and often strong enough to cause skin burns. Chemical fertilizers blaze a path through soil, destroying soil matter which would normally rot into a rich source of nutrients, and killing the microbes and other life that would achieve this. While chemical fertilizers cause the release of minerals from rocks in the soil, the microbes and mycorrhiza fungi disappear, making the released minerals unavailable to the plants. The same destructive process occurs with acid rain.

The combination of chemical fertilizer and pesticide use produces apparently healthy crops. The illusory appearance of large, good-looking fruits and vegetables masks the reality of severely compromised plant immunity brought about by inadequate nutrition. Nature would normally see to it that inferior plant life would not survive, but modern chemical treatments remove the fungi, insects and other life forms designed to carry out nature's work. Eventually, however, extreme natural conditions such as drought or frost reveal the serious inherent weaknesses of plants and soils treated with artificial fertilizers and we have farming disasters.

GOOD TRACE MINERALS DOWN, TOXIC ELEMENTS UP

Feed soil superphosphate fertilizer and crops grown on it will develop high levels of the toxic trace element cadmium. This has been known since work in the 1920s by soil scientist Dr. G. H. Earp-Thomas. Studies of trace elements show that under certain conditions toxic minerals can displace their beneficial cousins. Cadmium and essential zinc are good examples. This applies in the human body and soil alike. A plant growing in unbalanced soil containing high levels of cadmium will take up the toxic mineral in preference to zinc, actually blocking the plant's ability to absorb that essential element. The probable result for humans is an increase in uptake of cadmium, with its unfortunate ability to interfere with processes in the body that normally use zinc. The fact that Americans tend to be deficient in zinc owes much to this scenario.

The cadmium-zinc problem is only one of several examples. Where lead is present in high levels and calcium and magnesium are low, the body will take up lead instead of calcium and magnesium. This is a double whammy! The body is deprived of an essential mineral *and* poisoned with a toxic mineral.

Earp-Thomas also found that in the presence of too little sulfur a plant may take up toxic levels of selenium, and that chemical fertilizers high in phosphate will block the uptake of boron, a trace mineral increas-

ingly accepted as essential. Studies have shown that
boron decreases the loss of calcium and magnesium.
Boron is also thought to be involved in the production
of vitamin D and the synthesis of hormones, including estrogen.

It's important to remember that handy nutrition tables listing the amounts of vitamins and minerals in
foods can only serve as rough guides. They cannot tell
you, for example, if produce was grown in a mineral-
balanced soil or a polluted soil. Nor can they give
any indication of naturally occurring variations such as
selenium deficiency in high-rainfall areas of the U.S.
Chromium, iodine and selenium are three trace elements in particular that vary widely in soils from different geographic areas. What's more, many nutrition
tables have not been updated in twenty years or more!
In almost a century of practices which have continued
to rob the soil of vital mineral content, even one year
can make a difference to food values.

Studies show that natural farming produces foods
of greater nutritional value than those grown with artificial fertilizers. Organic foods are also far less contaminated by chemicals. A study from the Universities of
Maine and Vermont, published in 1987 in the *Journal
of Food Quality*, found much lower levels of calcium,
magnesium, beta-carotene and vitamin C in produce
grown using chemicals than in naturally grown vegetables. Several studies have shown that the protein content of grains is increased when natural farming
methods that maintain the mineral content of soil are
used. Minerals play a key role in the formation of
proteins. Molybdenum, for instance, is believed to be
required by bacteria which convert nitrogen into a
usable plant form. The resulting nitrates are used by
plants as the basis of proteins.

CHAPTER 4

Food and Water as Mineral Sources

Your best source of minerals is the food you eat every day. Taking supplements is important too. It's a form of health insurance which acknowledges that nobody's diet is perfect, and that a certain percentage of the food we eat will not be supplying us with the vitamins and minerals our bodies need for optimal health.

COOKING FOR MINERALS

How you cook your food can make all the difference between getting the minerals you need and becoming deficient in minerals. You could buy a fresh, crisp head of organic broccoli, wash and chop it carefully, together with tender, organic carrots and new potatoes then drop them lovingly into a pan full of boiling water for ten minutes. You could do all this and watch the trace elements and other nutrients go up in steam and down the pan. Alternatively, you could steam your veggies for just enough time to create succulent rather than soggy servings and preserve the nutrients. Stir-frying can seal in nutrients when done fast, hot, started with water and finished off with a small amount of olive oil. If you use frozen vegetables, steam them without thawing. Of course, frozen meat and fish should always be thawed thoroughly before cooking.

For meat and vegetable cooking, stewing can be healthful as long as meats are browned first and

193

drained of fat. Mineral and vitamin contents do leach out into broth, but will be consumed along with the finished stew.

Baking and roasting are both methods which cook using hot air. Bake or roast and you lose the fatty disadvantages of frying and the watery nutrient losses of boiling and steaming. Deep-frying only adds calories and potentially harmful chemicals. Cooking over charcoal and broiling bring the danger of contamination with chemicals in smoke from ignited fats. Broiling from above can help prevent this problem.

Microwave ovens should be reserved for rapid heating and defrosting. Long cooking with microwaves can change the chemistry of foods containing protein. Always use ceramic or glass containers for microwave preparation, as the heat causes chemicals to leach out from plastic and plastic wrap.

Foods lowest in fat content are foods richest in mineral nutrients. Selecting healthy foods and preparing them well prevents avoidable depletion of trace minerals, vitamins and other valuable nutrients.

WATER IS NOT THE MINERAL SOURCE IT USED TO BE

Running water is nature's primary delivery source of minerals. Its rushing, turbulent energy transports minerals from oceans and rocks to soil. It also leads to their existence in the highly available form of electrolytes. Research findings are now confirming that mineral absorption is highest when they are taken in dissolved form. Medical studies have shown this to be true of toxic minerals as well as dietary elements. One advantage that unpolluted, mineral-rich water has over foods is the absence of factors which can block mineral absorption. Such factors can be natural substances or chemical residues.

Ideally, drinking water should be an important source of trace elements. Unpolluted water from mountain and spring sources used to provide us with a range of beneficial minerals in a readily available form. Unfortunately, technology has created treated water for mass distribution that protects us from diseases such as cholera, but adds aluminum, chlorine and fluoride. Tap water is often also polluted with lead and copper from old plumbing. In high doses these substances compete with other important trace minerals for absorption.

In much of the industrialized world, municipal water treatment systems add aluminum to the water. Aluminum blocks other minerals in the body, it accumulates in the brain, liver, lungs and thyroid, and is a nerve poison in high amounts.

Chlorine, used to kill bacteria in water, is another toxic pollutant of tap water. In the gut, chlorine continues its sterilizing work, disturbing the balance of bacteria and potentially opening the door to an unfriendly overgrowth of organisms such as *Candida albicans*. Chlorine is also easily absorbed through the skin, especially in a hot shower when pores are open, adding to the body's overload.

Unless your water comes from a well that you check regularly for groundwater contaminants, I highly recommend that you purchase a water filter. A good one is expensive, but well worth the price for the health benefits, as you avoid chlorine, aluminum, benzene from petrochemical pollution, and many other potential hazards from treatment systems, industrial wastes and groundwater pollutants.

TRACE MINERALS AND THE FLUORIDATION CONTROVERSY

Many of what I call "health myths" have been sold to the American public in the name of profits. These myths creep in on the back of advertising, marketing, lobbying, political favors and kickbacks, and pretty soon they're taken as the gospel truth even though they're a pack of lies. There's the margarine-is-heart-healthy myth (the truth is that it has caused much more heart disease than it has prevented); there's the estrogen myth (it's more like the Grim Reaper than the Fountain of Youth), and there's the fluoride myth. I know, the common and seemingly irrefutable wisdom is that the number of cavities has been greatly decreased by the addition of fluoride to our drinking water and our toothpaste. I'm very sorry to say that it's not true, and that fluoride is most probably doing a great deal of harm.

Here's the story behind the story. During World War II we learned how to manufacture things from aluminum: airplanes, buildings and pots and pans, to name a few. We also greatly increased our production of chemical fertilizers. The down side of both these manufacturing processes was a byproduct called fluoride. Although fluoride is a trace mineral naturally occurring in our food, in anything but those trace amounts it's a more potent poison than arsenic. Disposing of the thousands of pounds of fluoride by-product became a major problem in American manufacturing. The manufacturers tried blowing it out their smokestacks, dumping it into rivers and burying it in the ground, but the immediate result was dead and deformed cows and other animals within miles of the smokestacks, rivers full of dead fish, and poisoned water aquifers. In fact its primary use was as a rat poison.

Finally, no doubt pushed by manufacturer's political pressure, the U.S. Public Health Service did a study claiming to show that one part per million of fluoride in water reduced tooth decay by 60 percent. Thus began the trickling of fluoride into our water supply.

The price of fluoride went up 1,000 percent almost overnight, and the problem of how to dispose of a potent toxin was solved. The practice of water fluoridation was further justified by more glowing studies claiming to show that communities using fluoridated drinking water had a much lower rate of tooth decay than those using unfluoridated water. The fluoride and cavity myth has been perpetuated by the fact that the rate of dental cavities has dropped steadily in the past thirty years, approximately the amount of time that our water has been fluoridated. So it must be good for us, right? Wrong.

The studies that were supposed to show how well fluoridated communities did are highly suspect. The original U.S. Public Health study on fluoridation was supposed to compare hundreds of communities, but the final study only included a few dozen, presumably those that fit the desired pro-fluoridation profile. And even those were flawed. For example, in the most widely cited study, two towns in Michigan were compared for dental cavities, but those children studied in the fluoridated community had higher incomes, received regular dental checkups, and agreed to brush their teeth twice a day. It wouldn't seem strange that they would have a lower rate of cavities, with or without fluoride!

"But," I hear you saying, "I had lots of cavities when I was a kid, and my kids hardly have any. It must be due to fluoride." Not so. In both fluoridated and unfluoridated areas in North America and Europe the decline in tooth decay has been the same for 30 years. This even holds true for entire countries in Europe that have not had fluoridated water or toothpaste. What has changed is that dental hygiene has improved, nutrition has improved, and access to dental care has improved. Studies do show a strong correlation between higher rates of tooth decay and lower economic status.

Japan and all of continental Europe either rejected the fluoride concept from the beginning or have stopped the practice. Most of Great Britain has also discontinued fluoridation, and Australia and New Zealand are in the process of reversing the trend. A 1994 study of virtually all New Zealand school children showed no benefit in dental health in fluoridated communities.

What's so bad about fluoride? There is good, solid evidence in eight reputable studies that fluoridated drinking water increases your risk of hip fractures by 20-40 percent. For a while it was thought that fluoride might actually help prevent osteoporosis. But long-term studies with hundreds of thousands of people proved the wisdom of checking things out thoroughly. There is a clear correlation between bone fractures and fluoridation. It turns out that while fluoride does create denser bone, it is poor-quality, structurally unsound bone that is actually more prone to fracture over time.

So much fluoride has been put into our water and toothpaste over the past 30 years that levels in our food chain are very high. Just by following a normal diet, the average person exceeds the recommended dose. Fluoride is a potent enzyme inhibitor that interferes with enzymes in the body, particularly in the lining of the intestines, causing stomach pain, gas and bloating. This enzyme-inhibiting effect also interferes with thyroid gland function. Some studies indicate that fluoride damages the immune system, leading to autoimmune disorders and arthritis. There is also evidence that communities with fluoridated water have a higher incidence of heart disease and higher rates of bone cancer in young men. Some 30 percent of children in fluoridated communities have fluorosis, a malformation of tooth enamel that causes discoloration (usually chalky white patches) and brittleness. This is a permanent change in the teeth that has also been associated with abnormal bone structure.

Advocates of putting fluoride in toothpaste and mouthwash argue that it is not swallowed, and therefore not ingested. However, fluoride is absorbed through the mucous membranes of the mouth, and young children do not have control over their swallowing reflex. There have been numerous reports of children poisoned by ingesting high levels of fluoride through school fluoride mouthwash programs, or fluoridated toothpastes full of sweeteners that kids want to swallow. (Please avoid both like the plague they are!) Who knows how many stomachaches in kids and adults alike have been caused by unknowingly ingesting too much fluoride?

While it is clear that fluoride can be helpful in the year or two when a child's adult teeth are growing in, there is absolutely no evidence that it is helpful before or after that time, and reams of evidence that it is harmful. A child's fluoride needs can be handled perfectly well by brushing with fluoride toothpaste for a few years. Other than that time of life, I recommend that you and your loved ones avoid fluoride in all forms, including toothpastes. This substance has crept into every link in our food chain, and the evidence is that even without fluoridated water and toothpaste we're getting a higher dose than is safe or recommended in our daily diets.

You can be thankful if you live in an unfluoridated community because it's not easy to get rid of fluoride in your tap water. Distillation and reverse osmosis are the only two reliable methods for removing fluoride. Other water filters may work at eliminating fluoride for a short period of time, but fluoride binds so strongly and quickly to filter materials such as charcoal, that the binding sites become fully occupied after a short time. If you are at a high risk for osteoporosis or heart disease, or if you have chronic digestive problems, I recommend you spend the money on a reverse osmosis water purification system.

REFINING FOODS EQUALS MINERAL ROBBERY

A better phrase than refined foods might be "nutrient-free." The obsession with convenience that has filled American lives since the '40s has brought increasingly dubious versions of food to TV trays across the land. When a food is refined, important parts of it are literally removed. White flour is produced by removing the outer husk of grains, consisting of the fibrous bran and germ, the part containing 95 percent of the nutrient value. The fiber is also removed from brown rice and whole sugar cane to give white variations of those foods. Advertising might lead us to believe that white sugar, rice and flour are "pure" foods. What they are is pure starch. "We need starch," you might say. This is true, but we also need essential minerals to aid in the digestion and processing of starch. The outer fiber of sugar and grains contains exactly the nutrients required to deal with the starch they surround.

Chromium found in the husk of grains is particularly needed in the processing of starch. Bran is itself fiber and contains other trace minerals like silicon and zinc as well as vitamin E and useful oils. Chromium is also found in unrefined sugar, where it is packaged with fiber and B complex vitamins. Fiber in products like unrefined flour and sugar provides bulk, acting as a check on excess consumption. Fiber also slows digestion and aids excretion of unwanted substances.

Pure starch taxes the body, as it stresses the pancreas and draws on stores of elements, especially chromium, needed for its digestion and absorption. What's more, as refined foods are processed, the body's acid/alkaline balance shifts toward acid. As the body works to restore its chemical balance it has to call even more on its mineral reserves. In this way, refining foods not only undersupplies but depletes trace minerals. Depletion is bad enough, but an additional result of eating only the inner core of rice and wheat grains is increased uptake of the element cadmium, which can accumulate to toxic levels. Cadmium is found largely in the central, starchy part of wheat and rice grains.

Unrefined wheat and rice are also packaged with zinc, mainly as part of their germ and bran. Zinc is absorbed by the body in preference to the toxic element, cadmium. Take away enough zinc and the cadmium is absorbed instead. White rice, white bread, white flour—all such refined products leave the door open to excess consumption of cadmium, which can inhibit the uptake of iron and block production of vitamin D.

Eating fresh, whole foods is like fitting the right keys into the locks of the body. Foods precooked, processed or refined in any other way may pick the locks of digestion and energy production, but they can damage them at the same time. Leave the convenience, fast and snack foods on the shelves and stick to whole, unrefined foods to keep your systems topped up with trace mineral levels and functioning smoothly.

"ENRICHED" FOODS ARE MINERAL POOR

U.S. law requires the addition of iron sulfate wherever iron and other minerals are removed during the processing of foods. Iron is an essential trace mineral with several valuable roles, particularly in the transportation of oxygen by the blood. I suppose the intention of this law is positive, but in practice it's almost useless, because iron sulfate is a form of iron that is not particularly well absorbed. In addition, absorption of the added iron in enriched food made with white flour or rice is likely to be blocked by other food additives or cadmium. Cadmium as an iron blocker is made available by the incidental removal of zinc during refining.

Does this make any sense to you? Iron is removed from foods, then replaced in questionable form, facing obstacles to its absorption. It is the same story or worse for other nutrients. More than thirty nutrients are removed from white, bleached flour. Four are added back, creating an "enriched" product. Ironically, the extracted nutrients are sold as animal feeds! To add insult to injury, manufacturers charge more for refined products sprayed with added nutrients. The only difference between one refined cereal and another can be sprayed-on vitamins and a higher price.

"Enriching" foods is nutritional nonsense. It plays havoc with the natural balances of trace elements established in foodstuffs. As seen with soil, mineral imbalances are perpetuated and worsened as nutrients are absorbed. The body has to scramble to provide minerals needed simply to digest foods robbed of their natural content, and it is not replenished. The selective replacement of a few nutrients ignores the fact that many work best when packaged with others that have not been restored.

Tinkering with the content of foods might pay the manufacturers, but it does not pay consumers in nutritional terms. Stay naturally enriched with trace minerals and other essential nutrients by steering clear of technologically "improved" food.

FIBER IS GOOD, BUT TOO MUCH IS NOT GOOD

Fiber is a perfect example of why moderation will keep you healthy in almost every aspect of your life. Fiber has been shown to be extremely important in the prevention of degenerative diseases including colitis, diverticulosis, ulcers and some cancers. Important minerals are packaged in the fiber around the energy-supplying starch in foods like rice and wheat. The body is adapted to absorb nutrients parceled in this way when they are consumed as part of a balanced diet.

The vast majority of Americans eat too many refined foods and don't get enough fiber. But too much isn't healthy either. Take in too much, and it will strip out trace elements and other nutrients. Fiber is largely indigestible and passes quickly out of the gut. Its ability to bind with toxins and other waste products is beneficial, in moderation. This ability simply extends too far when fiber levels are too high. It is highly unlikely that anyone will get too much fiber from the food they eat; most often the culprit is a fiber laxative or stimulant such as Metamucil (which is just psyllium with added colorings and sweeteners—the real thing is much, much cheaper and healthier).

If you're taking a fiber supplement such as psyllium, I recommend you take it first thing in the morning, at least half an hour before breakfast. This way it can stimulate and clean your digestive tract without taking nutrients with it. For the same reason, it's smart to take supplements at least an hour or two after taking a fiber supplement.

CHAPTER 5

Medicines and Mineral Depletion

I'll bet that when you take an antacid or an antibiotic, it never occurs to you that you could be creating a mineral deficiency or imbalance, but many, many over-the-counter (OTC) and prescription drugs interfere with mineral balance.

Some medications reduce mineral absorption, others cause minerals to be excreted in the urine in higher than normal quantities. Total intake of nutrients can change, too, as some drugs cause changes in appetite. In addition, the way a nutrient is used in the body can be altered by medications.

It is ironic that by disrupting nutrient uptake medications meant to heal the body can weaken it. One of the systems most impacted is the immune system, which requires vitamins and minerals for full protection against illness. A lack of nutrients may well lie behind a gap in the body's defenses which allows infection to take hold in the first place. Poor diet puts patients, particularly children and the elderly, at great risk from nutritional interference by drugs, especially if usage is long-term.

Research on drug and trace mineral interactions is sparse, but remember—wherever major minerals such as calcium, potassium and magnesium are lost, it's very likely that trace minerals are also being depleted.

Antacids are not a good source of calcium even though they may contain a great deal of it. In spite of advertising meant to convince you that stomach acid is your enemy, the truth is that heartburn and indigestion are most often caused by a *lack* of hydrochloric acid (HCl). Insufficient HCl leads to stomach churning and the fermentation of undigested food, which cause the food to be "urped" back up, burning the esophagus as it goes.

Taking antacids weakens or neutralizes acids for about an hour, relieving the symptoms, but often causing rebound heartburn or indigestion as the stomach tries to make up for the stomach acid it doesn't have by working overtime. In fact, in the long run, antacids will make heartburn and indigestion worse.

Antacids are advertised as being a good source of calcium, but this is misleading. The aluminum and magnesium in most antacids tend to bind with phosphate, which can result in calcium *depletion*! Weakened stomach acids cannot soften minerals, including calcium, arriving in the stomach. Minerals taken in are unlikely to be absorbed, and will almost certainly be excreted. The fact is that antacids can actually block calcium absorption and also tend to block iron absorption.

Some antacids deliver large amounts of compounds of aluminum, a trace element which can block mineral absorption and in large amounts can cause harm to the nervous system. Avoid taking antacids with citrus foods or drinks, as these increase the amount of aluminum absorbed. Aluminum hydroxides are the worst antacid culprits for blocking mineral absorption.

Used in too great amounts or for too long, antacids can produce vitamin and mineral deficiencies. If they do become necessary for extreme conditions, such as a true excess of HCl, their nutrient-blocking effects are lessened by taking them between meals or at night.

Most often I recommend that people with chronic heartburn and indigestion try taking betaine hydrochloride tablets before meals to aid digestion. Even simpler, just a warm glass of water with a tablespoon of apple cider vinegar can stimulate digestive juices and provide an acidic environment.

As an aside, please don't turn to the H2 blockers such as Tagamet, Pepcid and Zantac for heartburn and indigestion. They have a long list of side effects, and block the absorption of vitamin B12, which can cause symptoms of senility. Making these powerful drugs available over the counter is one of the most irresponsible actions the FDA has ever taken.

Antibiotics can be a powerful weapon against infection, but unfortunately they cannot distinguish between friend or foe. Antibiotics wipe out beneficial bacteria along with those causing harm. Take antibiotics and you will, for example, also destroy bacteria in the gut which produce the B-complex vitamin biotin. Mineral disruption can occur with the antibiotic Neomycin, which interferes with the absorption of calcium, iron, and potassium, as well as vitamin B12.

Some antibiotics interfere with the absorption of minerals, and the minerals interfere with the absorption of the antibiotic as well. Tetracycline blocks the absorption of dietary minerals by interacting with calcium, iron, magnesium and zinc, and taking these supplements will also block the action of the antibiotic.

Antibiotics known as quinolones will block the absorption of calcium, iron and zinc, and these minerals can also block the action of the antibiotic. Mineral supplements should be taken at least two hours away from tetracycline and the quinolones. Do not take antacids at the same time as these antibiotics either, because the calcium and magnesium may block their action.

As a general rule, problems with nutrient absorption end when the course of antibiotics ends. It is not advisable to take antibiotics for longer than about two weeks.

Anticonvulsants such as carbamazepine, phenobarbital, phenytoin and primidone block adequate production of vitamin D in the body. A lack of vitamin D leads the body to draw on calcium from bones instead of from dietary uptake. This is why long-term use of anticonvulsants can result in bone disorders. Another possible contributory factor in bone deformities caused by anticonvulsants is a lowering of blood and tissue levels of the trace mineral copper. Levels of zinc are also seen to drop over the long term when these drugs are used, compromising, among other functions, tissue formation and the immune system.

Antidepressants such as Fluoxetine, amoxapine, doxepin, imipramine and lithium carbonate may dampen the appetite and therefore indirectly cause nutrient deficiencies. Side effects such as abdominal cramps, diarrhea, dry mouth, nausea, and vomiting can occur with these types of drugs and with anti-anxiety medications like Librium and Valium. These symptoms can impair the absorption of nutrients. Long-term use of diazepam, for example, can disturb the balance of magnesium and calcium and increase the risk of bone disorders such as osteoporosis. Lithium disrupts copper absorption and may lead to a deficiency with long-term use.

Arthritis medications such as D-penicillamine can cause serious nutrient deficiencies, including mineral loss. Some of its side effects include an altered sense of taste, diarrhea, intestinal and digestive fluid problems, nausea, sores of the mouth and tongue, and vomiting, all of which can cause a loss of minerals. D-penicillamine reduces absorption of the trace element zinc, producing signs of clinical deficiency such as hair loss and skin changes. The drug binds to zinc and iron as well as other dietary minerals.

Aspirin can cause small amounts of blood to be lost in the stomach, and taking it regularly over a long period of time could result in enough blood loss to cause iron deficiency. I don't recommend that you take iron supplements, I recommend you avoid taking aspirin long-term! The pain killer indomethacin has the same problem.

Cholesterol-lowering drugs such as cholestyramine and colestipol lower the body's stores of iron as well as fat-soluble vitamins such as vitamins A, E and K, which are all protective against heart disease.

Corticosteroids such as cortisone and Prednisone are used to treat many illnesses, including arthritis and autoimmune diseases. They are also prescribed for skin problems, blood and eye disorders and asthma. Researchers conducted a study of 24 asthmatics using cortisone-type drugs and found the zinc levels were 42 percent lower than in patients not treated with corticosteroids.

Diuretics, frequently used in the treatment of high blood pressure and heart failure, can cause minerals to be lost in urine. Their effect is strongest with the beneficial minerals calcium, potassium and magnesium, but they also deplete the trace minerals iodine and zinc. Long-term diuretic use is definitely not encouraged. High blood pressure should always be vigorously treated first with lifestyle changes such as weight loss, exercise and a diet of nutrient-rich whole foods.

Laxatives turn nutrients into whistle-stop tourists of the intestine. Before they've had even a chance to inspect stomach or intestinal tract linings, nutrients are whisked away by laxatives. Even when nutrients do get to pause, laxatives like senna, and bisocodyl (Dulcolax) and phenolphthalein can interfere with the intestinal lining, possibly reducing nutrient uptake.

Mineral oil used as a laxative prevents absorption of vitamins A and D. Any laxative taken to excess can flush out large amounts of potassium, which can cause heart problems and muscle weakness.

Oral contraceptives tend to increase the levels of some vitamins and minerals, including copper, which in excess can cause a decrease in blood levels of iron and zinc. Studies have shown this type of medication can also lead to an increase in iron levels, possibly due to decreased menstrual flow.

Alcohol and tobacco. Alcohol is one our worst vitamin and mineral robbers. It depletes iron, selenium, zinc and magnesium, in addition to many other important nutrients. It also reduces the intake of minerals and nutrients in general by causing loss of appetite. Alcohol reduces absorption by damaging the lining of the small intestine and causes urinary loss of minerals. Alcoholic drinks like wine and whiskey are also relatively high in the toxic element cadmium, which is taken up in greater quantities when zinc levels are low.

While a glass of wine with dinner may be beneficial, tobacco is not suitable in any quantity! And remember that the harmful nutritional effects of tobacco extend to people breathing second-hand smoke. This is true especially because nonsmokers breathe in the unfiltered smoke which contains more poisons than the smoke breathed through a filtered cigarette. The trace element zinc and many other nutrients drop to low levels in smokers, impairing the immune system as well as the ability to detoxify the poisons being absorbed. Low zinc levels lead to a greater uptake and absorption of the trace element cadmium, which happens to be one of the toxins in tobacco smoke. Pregnant women who smoke are more likely to give birth to zinc-deficient babies.

CHAPTER 6

Keeping the Trace Minerals in Balance

Wouldn't life be a lot simpler if nutrition were only a matter of opening our mouths and pouring down a liquid super-food? Well, yes, but *we'd* be simpler, too, possibly drifting as a single cell in the ocean. As complex organisms, we have complex nutritional needs which are automatically supplied by foods in their natural forms. For example, whole-wheat bread brings the elements needed to digest it, and fruit delivers fast energy supported by the nutrients required to process it. Yet the production of our foods has to be literally rooted in properly balanced soils to ensure that nutrients blend as nature intended and health requires. Trace mineral interactions are examples of the way partnerships of nutrients abound. Research is increasingly showing the importance of nutrients in combination, which is powerfully demonstrated by the effects of trace minerals in and out of balance.

THE BODY WORKS TO CREATE OPTIMUM TRACE MINERAL LEVELS

The body is actually designed to maintain healthy levels of many trace minerals and hundreds of other biologically active chemicals. It performs constant, subtle adjustments in a wonderful, automatic effort to maintain balance, also known as homeostasis. (I think this word is misleading, because *stasis* means standing or stopping, and maintaining balance in the body is one of the most active processes I can think of.)

Excess trace elements are removed by preventing their absorption or triggering their excretion. Excretion occurs through feces, urine and sweat. Hair can also be a minor route of excretion for metallic trace minerals. Essential trace elements are nontoxic except in large amounts, and the body can temporarily tolerate a wide range between the highest and lowest levels associated with health. At low levels, the body can survive with an amount of a trace element sufficient for growth and maintenance, but insufficient for optimum function.

Mineral balance can be interfered with and overwhelmed, leading to inadequate or excess absorption. Normally the maintenance of optimum levels of trace minerals is affected by dietary consumption.

The intestines can reject excess amounts of trace minerals just as the kidneys can excrete them. However, both organs can only handle so much of any trace mineral. If that amount is exceeded, the body accumulates the mineral to poisonous levels.

TOXIC ELEMENTS CAN TAKE THE PLACE OF TRACE MINERALS

All elements, even oxygen, can become toxic at high enough levels. Extremely poisonous chemicals, such as mercury, are simply those that have toxic effects in very small amounts. Fortunately for the human race, nature has locked away many of the substances which are harmful in low amounts. Humans, however, have been uncovering them at increasing rates, mining uranium and other heavy metals and minerals. We are also exposed to unprecedented levels of lead through car exhaust, and cadmium through poor agricultural processes. This has increased the need for trace elements required to help protect the body and process noxious chemicals. It has also led to a greater chance that toxic chemicals may be absorbed instead of essential trace elements.

Essential trace minerals belong to different families of elements which include toxic cousins. Just as with plants, if not enough of a particular trace element is present, the body will take up its nearest available cousin. Illness can be caused, for example, when cadmium displaces zinc, changing or inactivating enzymes. Disease conditions can occur when insufficient iodine causes the thyroid gland to take up sodium fluoride instead. Iodine pills were issued by the Polish government after the nuclear disaster of Chernobyl in 1986. This was to try to prevent an uptake of radioactive iodine in place of essential iodine.

The best prevention of toxic element uptake is to avoid exposure by buying organic foods and living in an unpolluted environment. A healthy diet also protects you from harmful elements by maintaining trace element levels, filling any gaps a toxic cousin might fit. Optimum levels of trace elements also aid the body's detoxifying mechanisms.

HOW ESSENTIAL TRACE ELEMENTS INTERACT

The interaction of several trace minerals and other nutrients requires a cautious and intelligent approach to supplementation. The human body is geared to receive nature's own balanced recipes of nutrients that exist in individual foods. Ideally, trace elements and other nutrients should be readily available from whole food sources without major concerns about their correct proportions or partners. Sadly, a compromised and polluted environment leads to an unbalanced uptake of nutrients and unnatural toxins. This generates a need for wisely chosen supplements and diet. Awareness of the types of stress which use up trace minerals helps to promote use of supplements at the right time. Supplies of zinc, for example, are run down with infection, and iron will be lost with extensive bleeding.

A good general rule is to avoid taking higher-than-recommended doses of any one mineral without taking into account the effect it will have on other minerals, especially when taking them long-term. Trace mineral interactions include the following:

Cobalt and molybdenum. Molybdenum antagonizes cobalt.

Cobalt and iodine. Cobalt antagonizes iodine.

Copper and molybdenum. Molybdenum may alter copper absorption, but copper is also believed to work against molybdenum.

Copper and selenium. Copper is believed by some investigators to be a selenium antagonist, probably competing for absorption.

Iron and magnesium carbonate. Excessive magnesium carbonate could reduce the absorption of iron. (Note: Magnesium carbonate is not a good magnesium supplement since it is not easily absorbed.)

Iron, copper, manganese and zinc. Take too much of one and you may cause a deficiency in another of these trace minerals, creating an increased risk of infection and other diseases. These elements compete for absorption in the small intestine. When in balance, copper enhances the absorption and utilization of iron. Zinc in particular competes against copper for absorption.

CHAPTER 7

Food Sources of Essential Trace Minerals

The food values found in tables do not account for variations caused by climate, geology and time of harvesting, or those caused by chemical farming. However, they do provide basic information about which foods are usually comparatively high in certain trace minerals and other nutrients. It's a good idea to hedge against depletion of nutrients in any one food by eating a range that in theory supplies the content you are looking for.

Boron. Good sources are fruits and vegetables.

Chromium. Good sources are black pepper, thyme, cheese, lean meat, and whole grain cereals.

Cobalt. Good sources are meats and other foods of animal origin.

Copper. Good sources are shellfish, especially oysters, avocado, fish, poultry, dark green leafy vegetables, cooked soybeans, dried peas and other legumes, nuts, bananas and other fruits, whole-grain bread and cereals and cooked carrots.

Iodine. Good sources include iodized salt, seafood and seaweed.

Iron. Good sources (all better than spinach) include red meats, brewer's yeast, kelp, lima beans, chickpeas, duck, shellfish, molasses, wheat bran, parsley and apricots.

Manganese. Good sources are whole grains, nuts, shellfish and milk. Given soil that is not too alkaline, fruit and green vegetables can be moderate sources of manganese.

Molybdenum. Good sources are whole grains, dark green leafy vegetables, peas, beans, and milk. Crops grown on depleted soil can have molybdenum levels up to 500 times lower than plants grown on soil rich in this mineral.

Selenium. Good sources are brewer's yeast, broccoli, cabbage, celery, cucumbers, fish, garlic, whole grains, mushrooms, and poultry. However, selenium levels vary greatly in soils. As a general rule, soils in the Western states are lower in selenium than soils in Eastern ones.

Zinc. Good sources are fish, meat, oysters, and whole grains.

KELP

Kelp, a seaweed, is an excellent source of minerals. It contains 23 minerals, the most important of which are present in the percentages shown:

Iodine	0.15-0.20%	Magnesium	0.76%
Calcium	1.20	Sulfur	0.93
Phosphorus	0.30	Copper	0.0008
Iron	0.10	Zinc	0.0003
Sodium	3.14	Manganese	0.0008
Potassium	0.63		

Vitamins present in kelp are: vitamin B2, niacin, choline and carotene. Algenic acid is also present. This remarkable food contains more vitamins and minerals than any other substance. All these nutrients have been assimilated by the growing plant.

Kelp, because of its natural iodine content, acts to normalize the thyroid gland. Therefore, thin people with thyroid trouble may gain weight by using kelp, and obese people with thyroid trouble may lose weight.

If you need a good supply of highly absorbable minerals, try taking kelp supplements.

CHAPTER 8

The *Good* Trace Minerals from A to Zinc

Minerals work in partnership with hormones, enzymes, amino acids and vitamins. They are required to build and maintain the structure of the body. They are involved in the breakdown of food during digestion, and some are instrumental in maintaining fluid balance inside cells. Those that are currently considered essential for human nutrition are calcium, phosphorus, iron, potassium, selenium, and magnesium. In reality, however, many more minerals are needed to maintain optimal health. Chromium, cobalt, copper, zinc and manganese are important in their own right, even though we only require them in very small amounts.

Unless you are trying to correct a specific nutritional deficiency under the supervision of a health care professional, minerals should only be taken in the recommended doses, as an excess can cause just as many problems as a deficiency.

Let's take a closer look at the trace minerals you should be getting in your daily vitamin program.

BORON

Boron is a trace mineral that helps retard bone loss and works with calcium, magnesium and vitamin D to help

221

prevent osteoporosis (brittle bones). Some studies suggest that a boron deficiency may aggravate arthritis and other degenerative joint conditions. Boric acids and borates have been used medicinally for centuries as disinfectants and to treat burns.

As I mentioned earlier in the book, we tend to be deficient in boron, because the use of superphosphate fertilizers blocks its uptake by plants.

According to boron researcher Forrest H. Nielsen of the Department of Agriculture's Grand Forks Human Nutrition Research Center, calcium cannot be properly metabolized without boron. He fed a low-boron diet (less than 0.32 milligram per day) to five men, five postmenopausal women on bone-preserving estrogen therapy, and four postmenopausal women not on estrogen, for 63 days. Then, for the next 49 days, they continued on the low-boron diet, but added a daily 3-mg supplement of boron.

On the low-boron diet, blood levels of calcium decreased, along with other nutrients that affect bone health. When boron was added back in, all these measures improved, and copper levels improved as well.

You can take 1-3 milligrams of boron daily—not more than that—if you are at risk for osteoporosis. Otherwise, you can get boron in a healthy diet. Boron is abundant in pears, apples and grapes, and is also found in nuts, green, leafy vegetables and legumes such as soy beans.

CHROMIUM

Chromium is one of our most important trace minerals, and one of the most depleted. It works with insulin in the metabolism of sugar and helps the body utilize protein and fats. Taken in conjunction with exercise, chromium helps the body burn off fat more efficiently. It is best to take chromium in the form of chromium picolinate. Chromium also helps prevent and lower high blood pressure.

Recent studies suggest that chromium may help athletes by regulating the body's use of glycogen during exercise. In one study, weight lifters using chromium supplements had greater muscle and weight gains than a group given a placebo. In another study, chromium supplements lowered blood cholesterol levels.

It is also very important to those with blood sugar and insulin imbalances, such as diabetics. Chromium is necessary for glucose to enter the cells, so it is essential in the efficient burning of carbohydrates. In fact, a chromium deficiency may cause adult-onset diabetes, especially in older people.

I know the people who make those awful bottled "natural" fruit drinks and teas aren't going to like me for saying this, but I suspect that the steep rise in our consumption of high-fructose corn syrup has contributed to the rise in diabetes by depleting chromium. (As our consumption of high-fructose corn syrup has risen 250 percent in the past 15 years, our rate of diabetes has increased approximately 45 percent in about the same time period.) According to studies done at the Agriculture Department's Human Nutrition Resource Center, fructose consumption causes a drop in chromium, as well as raising "bad" LDL cholesterol and triglycerides, and impairing immune system function.

According to researchers, giving people with elevated blood sugar a chromium supplement will result in a significant drop in blood sugar in 80 to 90 percent of those people.

Chromium may also be important for skin health. In a study reported in *Medical Hypotheses*, when nine patients with acne were given two teaspoons daily of high-chromium yeast containing 400 micrograms of chromium, their acne rapidly cleared up.

Please don't be scared away from chromium by recent media reports about it. Taking chromium picolinate supplements of 100 to 600 mcg daily is not the same as exposing hamster cells in a test tube to 5,000 to 6,000 times that dose every day, nor is it the same as factory workers breathing chromium dust.

Most Americans are actually deficient in chromium, and at the recommended doses it is very safe and very effective in helping stabilize blood sugar as well as helping burn fat during exercise and producing lean muscle tissue.

You can take 200 mcg of chromium daily, depending on your needs. Food sources of chromium include brewer's yeast, whole grains, nuts, molasses and cheese.

COBALT

Cobalt is a component of vitamin B12, and as such is a stimulant to the production of red blood cells, and is necessary for normal cell growth and healthy nerve tissue. A deficiency of cobalt/B12 can cause anemia. Although a deficiency of cobalt is rare, it can occur in vegetarians, since cobalt is mainly found in meat and shellfish in the form of vitamin B12. Cobalt can also replace other trace minerals in enzyme reactions, and is part of the enzyme action involved in forming some antioxidants.

COPPER

Copper and zinc balance each other in the body, and a deficiency of one can cause an excess of the other. Copper is necessary for absorption and utilization of iron and the formation of red blood cells.

Copper works as a catalyst in the formation of red blood cells and is present in the hemoglobin molecule. It also plays a role in maintaining the skeletal system. Copper is essential before iron can be utilized and is necessary to prevent anemia. It is an important partner to vitamin C in the synthesis of collagen. You don't usually need to add copper to your diet. An excess can cause hair loss, insomnia, irregular menses and depression.

FLUORIDE

Fluoride helps protect teeth from decay and may help protect against osteoporosis. Too much causes discolored teeth and continued overuse of it may lead to bone fractures, abnormal bony growths, heart disease and digestive disorders. Most Americans get excessive fluoride in their normal diet, just by drinking tap water, sodas, and other commercial products made with fluoridated water. I don't recommend that you supplement fluoride in your diet. See page 21 for more about the fluoridation controversy.

IODINE

As far back as Hippocrates, physicians have known that something in seaweed and seafood prevents goiter, an enlargement of the thyroid gland. Iodine is the key component in a thyroid hormone called thyroxin, and a lack of it causes the thyroid gland to enlarge. Since the thyroid regulates our metabolism—how fast we use energy—it is an essential trace mineral. And yet, it is a trace mineral found in the sea, and rarely inland. Many inland areas of the world are still deficient in iodine and suffer from diseases relating to improper thyroid function.

Iodine is necessary for proper growth, and promotes healthy hair, nails, skin and teeth. A deficiency of iodine in pregnant women can cause retardation in their children, and children deficient in it may become retarded. A deficiency of vitamin A can make iodine deficiency even worse.

Iodine deficiency can be caused by eating too many vegetables in the cabbage family (kale, cauliflower, turnips) without a sufficient intake of iodine. A substance in these vegetables blocks the uptake of iodine. Disease conditions can occur when insufficient iodine causes the thyroid gland to take up sodium fluoride instead.

Sufficient iodine levels also confers some protection against radiation damage, as a lack of it will cause the thyroid to take up the radioactive trace elements instead. As mentioned earlier, it was for this reason that the Polish government distributed iodine pills after the Chernobyl nuclear disaster.

An oversupply of iodine can cause or aggravate acne in adolescents. Some researchers speculate that this is caused when the excess iodine is excreted through the pores, irritating the skin.

Seafoods are very high in iodine, and it is added to most table salt. Kelp is a good source of natural iodine. You should be getting 150 mcg or 0.15 mg of iodine daily as part of your food or in your multivitamin. Pregnant and nursing women should be getting 175-200 mcg daily.

IRON

Iron is required in the manufacture of hemoglobin, a component of blood, and helps carry oxygen in the blood. It works with many enzymes in biochemical reactions in the body, and to be used efficiently must also have copper, cobalt, manganese and vitamin C. B-complex vitamins such as B1, B6, biotin, folic acid and B12, all work with iron to produce rich red blood.

Women need more iron than men because of the

loss of blood during the menstrual cycle, and their need for iron is increased during pregnancy and breast feeding.

In excess, iron is not efficiently excreted from the body. It can accumulate in tissue and become toxic. Recent research has shown that excessive amounts of iron in the tissues raises the risk of heart disease. Some researchers theorize that part of the reason a woman's risk of heart disease increases after menopause is that she is not losing iron every month during menstruation. Although iron is an essential mineral, it is important not to take too much iron in supplement form. A deficiency can cause a specific disease called iron deficiency anemia.

The most noticeable warning sign of anemia, a sign of iron deficiency, is fatigue. If you are getting plenty of rest, but still feel tired and lacking in energy, your body could be telling you that you are becoming anemic. The hair, skin and nails also show the effects of anemia. The skin tends to wrinkle more. Fingernails and toenails become brittle and break easily, and become tender. Hair becomes dry and lacks luster. Skin color becomes paler, even pasty and gray. The mouth and tongue begin to feel sore and tender.

Since the most available sources of absorbable iron are meat, vegetarians are at a greater risk of becoming iron-deficient.

Sufficient iron levels are essential for top athletic performance. Since iron plays a role in delivering oxygen to the muscles, iron-poor blood can cause less efficient use of muscles and fatigue. Studies have shown that women athletes in particular may benefit from iron supplements, even when iron levels test as normal. A study of high-school cross-country runners found 45 percent of the female runners and 17 percent of the male runners had low iron levels during the competitive season. Another study of 100 female college students showed that 31 percent had iron deficiency. The population most susceptible to iron deficiency is young women who are dieting to keep their weight down, and also exercising strenuously. For young athletes, keeping the body well stocked with iron can improve endurance and keep red blood cells optimally healthy.

Iron supplements can cause constipation, diarrhea, nausea and poor absorption of zinc. Your best bet is to eat plenty of iron-rich foods and keep iron supplements low. In fact, I don't recommend iron supplements except for young women and possibly pregnant women as needed, unless blood tests show low iron levels. Most iron deficiency anemia can be cured by proper diet. If you need iron supplementation, 10 mg daily is a reasonable amount to take. If you want to take more, please do so under the guidance of a health care professional who can measure your iron levels.

LITHIUM

Lithium is a trace mineral only recently studied, and is not needed in significant enough amounts in the body to be supplemented. However, lithium has been used successfully for years to treat manic depression, now known as bipolar mood disorder. It is a treatment that must be used with care, because it interacts with other substances, and can cause kidney damage and death if it accumulates to a toxic level.

Some researchers have used lithium to successfully treat those attempting to withdraw from alcohol, cocaine and other drugs.

The two most common side effects of lithium are weight gain and fatigue, which may be caused by reduced thyroid function, even though thyroid tests are normal. Lithium may also cause a deficiency of folic acid, which can increase the risk of heart disease and some cancers, and cause a deficiency of vitamin B12. A report from the National Institutes of Health suggests that taking the B vitamin inositol with lithium may reduce the side effects.

Lithium also replaces sodium when there is a sodium deficiency, which can upset the delicate balance of fluid in the cells, causing edema, nausea and vomiting.

Many arthritis and pain medications interfere with lithium excretion and can cause a toxic buildup. These include aspirin, ibuprofen (Advil, Motrin), naproxen (Aleve), and indomethacin (Indocin). Both the thiazide diuretics (furosemide, bumetanide) and the potassium-sparing diuretics (spironolactone, triamterene) used to treat high blood pressure can also raise lithium levels dangerously. The same is true of the heart drugs known as ACE inhibitors, such as captopril, enalapril and quinapril. The anticonvulsant carbamazepine (Tegretol) can make lithium more effective in some people, but in others can cause toxicity.

I recommend that you use lithium only under the guidance of a health-care professional. If you are taking it and experience nausea, diarrhea, muscle weakness, call your doctor immediately.

MANGANESE

Manganese is another trace mineral that we're learning more about every day. It is an important trace mineral that activates numerous enzymes, and is related to proper utilization of vitamins B1, E and iron. Manganese is also involved with thyroid function, the central nervous system, and digestion of proteins. It increases levels of the antioxidant SOD (superoxide dismutase).

Very little manganese is stored in the body, making it an important mineral to include in a supplement

program. Too much manganese interferes with iron
absorption, and conversely, too much iron can reduce
manganese levels.

Although manganese deficiency is not well studied,
some of the symptoms of manganese deficiency are
middle ear problems, reduced fertility, retarded
growth and low blood sugar.

A study of trace metals conducted during autopsies
of 32 people, of whom 16 had blocked arteries,
showed that those with the heart disease had low copper and manganese levels in the damaged arteries.

Manganese plays a role in the breakdown of collagen, and a deficiency can cause dermatitis; it can reduce levels of "good" HDL cholesterol, and cause
bone loss and bone instability. A study of women with
osteoporosis showed that they had low manganese levels, and rodent studies indicate that it is a crucial mineral in the formation of strong, normal bone.

Researchers all over the world have reported success
in treating schizophrenia with manganese, and some
theorize that it plays an important role in stabilizing
nerve transmissions. It has also been used to treat seizures, and this may be connected to its important role
in the middle ear.

Manganese is one of the important trace minerals
removed when grains are refined. The prevalence of
nutrition-free refined foods in America has made manganese deficiency common. Since manganese competes with calcium, it should be taken separately as
a supplement.

I recommend that women at risk for osteoporosis
add 5-10 mg of manganese to their daily supplements,
and other adults include 2-5 mg daily.

MOLYBDENUM

This trace mineral was once considered toxic because
miners inhaling it became ill. However, we now know

that it is important to human health in very small quantities. It is used by blue-green algae and other plant life to turn nitrogen into a useable compound essential to all life, so its presence is foundational to life as we know it.

A deficiency of molybdenum has been linked to age-related cataracts and cancer of the stomach and esophagus. It is one of the trace elements necessary for the metabolism of iron, and it plays important roles in at least three enzyme systems having to do with the metabolism of fats, carbohydrates and proteins.

There is evidence that sufficient molybdenum is important to the formation of strong teeth, which makes sense since it is a component of tooth enamel, and it is vital to the normal development of the fetus.

Since molybdenum and copper compete with each other, an excess of one can cause a deficiency of the other. Excess sulfur can also cause a deficiency of molybdenum.

Molybdenum is one of the trace minerals stripped out of refined grains, and depleted from many soils. I recommend that you include 100-250 mcg of molybdenum in your daily vitamin intake.

SELENIUM

Selenium is a trace mineral found in very small amounts in the body. However, its role in maintaining our health is anything but small. I have been telling my readers about this mineral for 20 years. In 1957, Dr. Klaus Schwarz and Dr. C. M. Katz established that selenium is essential to life, even though it is needed in very small quantities, but it was not until 1990 that it was designated as a recommended dietary allowance (RDA) mineral. This means that your body must have this mineral daily. If we need selenium in such small amounts, why do we need to add it to our diets? White bread is one answer. Processing grain to produce white flour robs it of 75 percent of its selenium content.

Selenium could be called the "anticancer" mineral. Over and over again population studies have shown that people living in areas containing plenty of selenium in the soil have lower rates of cancer, and those living in areas with selenium-depleted soil have higher rates, especially of colon cancer.

Selenium is an antioxidant that also stimulates the immune system. A deficiency can lead to impaired immune function and reduced T-cell counts.

It works synergistically with vitamin E, each enhancing the actions of the other. Selenium is found in high concentrations in semen, and men seem to need more of this mineral than women. A selenium deficiency can cause dandruff, dry skin and fatigue, and may be associated with the development of cataracts.

Selenium is important in male hormone regulation and is found in large amounts in the prostate. Blood levels of both zinc and selenium are low in men who have prostate cancer. Men who live in areas where the soil is rich in selenium tend to have lower rates of prostate cancer.

Selenium is protective against heavy metal exposure, specifically to mercury, it is important in the formation of the antioxidant glutathione, and has been associated with reductions in heart disease.

Selenium also aids in keeping youthful elasticity to your tissues, can help alleviate hot flashes and other menopausal symptoms, and helps in the treatment and prevention of dandruff.

If you're over the age of 50 I suggest you supplement your diet with up to 200 mcg of selenium daily.

VANADIUM

Vanadium is a mineral mainly stored in our bones and fat. Although no human deficiency of vanadium has ever been identified, in test animals a deficiency caused impaired growth of teeth, bones and cartilage, thyroid changes, decreased overall growth, and fluid retention. This mineral can also be used to build up teeth, bones, cartilage and even muscle. It stimulates cell division, but also has anticarcinogenic properties.

A substance called vanadyl sulfate, which is derived from vanadium, is used to increase muscle growth and development, and appears to make muscles larger and denser more rapidly than would normally be the case.

Vanadyl sulfate is also very important in the treatment of diabetes. It helps insulin work more efficiently, and that may be why it also lowers cholesterol and triglyceride levels.

If you have diabetes, I don't recommend long-term high doses of vanadium, but you can use it to help stabilize your blood sugar, and then cut back. Try starting with 6 mg daily and work your way up to 100 mg daily until you get results. Once you begin having results, stay at that dose for up to three weeks and then taper back gradually to 6-10 mg daily.

Normally it is not necessary to include vanadium as a dietary supplement.

ZINC

Think of zinc as a traffic policeman, directing and overseeing the efficient flow of body processes, the maintenance of enzyme systems, and the integrity of our cells. It is a tiny but powerful catalyst which is absolutely essential for most body functions.

Zinc is a trace mineral found in the thyroid gland, hair, finger- and toenails, nervous system, liver, bones, pancreas, kidney, pituitary glands, blood and in the male reproductive fluid or semen. It is the prime element in male hormone production. Zinc is a constituent of insulin, which is necessary for the utilization of sugar. It also assists food absorption through the intestinal wall.

Zinc governs the contractility of our muscles, stabilizes blood, and maintains the relationship of acidity and alkalinity in the blood and other fluids. Zinc is essential for the synthesis of protein and in the action of many enzymes. A lack of zinc can cause increased fatigue, susceptibility to infection and injury and a slowdown in alertness and scholastic achievement.

Zinc exerts a normalizing effect upon the prostate and a lack of the mineral can produce testicular atrophy and prostate trouble. Zinc is necessary for the proper function of the prostate gland. In men, higher concentrations of this mineral are found in the prostate than anywhere else in the body. A recent study looked at zinc supplementation in young men, and found that when plasma zinc levels were low, there was a corresponding drop in testosterone. There have been many clinical studies showing that zinc supplementation can reduce the size of the prostate gland, along with troublesome symptoms.

Zinc supplements during pregnancy appear to promote an increase in birth weight. When you exercise vigorously, you lose a lot of zinc, so it's important for athletes to take a zinc supplement.

Most zinc available in foods is lost in processing. For example, 80 percent of the zinc in white bread is destroyed by processing. White spots or bands on the fingernails may indicate zinc deficiency.

Zinc supplements can be taken as lozenges, and in that form can cut down the length and severity of colds and flus, especially when combined with vitamin C.

Zinc is important in maintaining clear skin. Zinc stimulates antibody production to help fend off invading organisms on the skin surface. Some adolescent acne may be caused by a zinc deficiency.

As with all minerals, please don't take zinc in excess as it will cause other imbalances in your body. Zinc works best in combination with vitamin A, calcium and phosphorus.

I recommend that all men take up to 15-30 mg of zinc daily, and include zinc-rich foods in the diet such as oysters (well cooked please!), lamb chops and wheat germ. Pumpkin seeds are a good source of zinc.

Pregnant women and athletes can take 15-30 mg daily.

Everyone else should include 5-15 mg of zinc in their daily vitamin supplements.

CHAPTER 9

The *Bad* Trace Minerals and How to Avoid Them

The following trace minerals I have labeled as "bad" because, although they exist in the body in extremely small amounts, they can cause toxicity in minute doses, some as small as a few parts per million. Even the "good" trace minerals are only beneficial in very small amounts, and become toxic in large amounts. The toxic metals tend to accumulate in the body, increasing their potential for toxicity. Some can enter the brain, causing serious biochemical imbalances. Pollution by industrial wastes, car exhaust, farming with artificial fertilizers, pesticides and fungicides, copper and lead in pipes, polluted ground water, as well as cooking and eating utensils made of these substances, has created an environment where metal poisoning is common in the industrialized world.

It's easy to become frightened after reading about the pervasiveness of these metals in the environment and the extent of the damage they can do to the body, and there is certainly cause for concern and watchfulness. Your best ally is education; finding out what the sources of these metals are, and then avoiding them as best you can. A single exposure to toxic trace minerals is unlikely to cause serious illness unless it is a very large dose. Most poisoning occurs through small doses over time.

Exposure to toxic trace minerals can be insidious, because the symptoms may be generalized and not severe enough to warrant a visit to the doctor or proper blood testing by a doctor, yet be severe enough to cause chronic fatigue, headaches, dizziness and/or mental and emotional symptoms such as irritability, confusion, memory loss, hyperactivity and even violent behavior.

According to research reported by the American Society For Reproductive Medicine, air pollution with heavy metals may be an unsuspected cause of infertility. Exposure to cadmium, nickel, manganese and zinc at concentrations not high enough to be directly toxic can produce changes in sperm that cause infertility. Male infertility is increasing at an alarming rate. Some estimates put it at 1 percent per year. (Exposure to hormone-altering pesticides is also playing a role in male infertility.)

A balanced nutritious diet, drinking plenty of clean water, moderate exercise and a daily multiple vitamin will make a big difference in your body's ability to detox and clear out any overload of toxic minerals. Getting the "good" minerals in your daily vitamin regimen is particularly important because many of the toxic trace minerals replace good minerals such as calcium, iron and zinc.

ALUMINUM

Thanks to industrial pollution and the widespread use of aluminum in foods, medicines, municipal water treatment and cosmetics, people living in industrialized nations are exposed to much higher levels of this metal than is safe.

Although it is the third most abundant element in the earth's crust, aluminum is only found in very small amounts in plants and animals. Up to a point, our bodies are well equipped to safely excrete most of the aluminum we ingest. But in larger doses it becomes toxic, causing bone abnormalities, muscle weakness, loss of balance and coordination, memory loss and depression. Because aluminum interferes with the absorption of important minerals such as selenium, magnesium and calcium, its toxic effects can include the deficiency diseases caused by lack of these minerals.

The fact that aluminum's toxicity remains controversial has more to do with greed and politics than a lack of scientific research. Aluminum in excess is clearly a poison, but it is also the third most used metal product in the United States. This means that the aluminum lobbyists are well endowed and powerful enough to discourage government action that might decrease our exposure to aluminum.

Because aluminum is so pervasive in the environment, it pays to avoid it whenever possible, because even then you're likely to be getting regular overdoses of it.

Aluminum and Alzheimer's Disease

Although research into the connection between Alzheimer's disease and aluminum remains controversial, it is clear from half a dozen good population studies that those with higher levels of aluminum in their water supply have higher levels of Alzheimer's. Rats whose brains are injected with aluminum have symptoms similar to those of Alzheimer's. A Johns Hopkins University study found that those patients undergoing hemodialysis who had increased levels of aluminum also had decreased levels of cognitive brain function. The authors of that study theorized that aluminum may interfere with the brain's ability to use glucose, and thus its ability to produce important brain chemicals such as acetylcholine.

It may also be that some people have a genetic susceptibility to brain damage caused by a combination of factors, including aluminum. Whatever the cause or combination of causes, aluminum is clearly implicated in Alzheimer's disease, and for that reason alone I would recommend you avoid it.

Sources of Aluminum

One of the most pervasive sources of aluminum is simply industrial byproducts, blown out smokestacks, dumped into rivers and waste sites and trickling into our water aquifers. The secondary effect of industrial air pollution is acid rain, which contains high levels of aluminum which leaches through the soil into ground water over time.

Aluminum also enters water through municipal treatment plants because aluminum sulfate (alum) is used to clarify the water. To add insult to injury, there is some evidence that adding fluoride to the water makes the aluminum even more toxic by making it more difficult to excrete. Aluminum fluoride also crosses the blood-brain barrier more easily, exposing the brain to increased levels of both aluminum and fluoride. Ironically, the sodium fluoride pumped into America's water supplies is a waste product of aluminum manufacturing!

Aluminum is very commonly used in processed foods as an emulsifier, to prevent clumping, and to whiten ingredients. It is found in processed flours of all kinds, baking powder, processed fruits and vegetables, and table salt. There are literally dozens of variations on aluminum additives, but some of the more common ones you'll find on food labels are: alum, aluminum potassium sulfate, sodium aluminum phosphate, sodium silicon aluminate, aluminum calcium silicate, potassium alum, aluminum stearate and aluminum hydroxide. Suffice it to say that anything with the word aluminum in it counts.

Probably the next most common source of aluminum is antacids. Antacid users can easily consume 5 grams (5,000 mg) of aluminum per day. Since 150 mg a day is considered a safe level of aluminum consumption, antacids represent a major source of aluminum overdose. Indigestion and heartburn become more common as we age, and antacid use and abuse rises steeply in people over the age of 50. (See my book in this series, *Dr. Earl Mindell's What You Should Know About Fiber and Digestion,* for specifics on preventing and treating indigestion and heartburn naturally.) As we age, we accumulate heavy metals in our tissues, so throwing any additional burden on top of an already overloaded system may be pushing some senior citizens into symptoms of senility by blocking essential trace minerals such as selenium, and causing brain chemistry changes. Antacids also interfere with the absorption of nutrients, so I recommend that you avoid them except for occasional use, and then use antacids that don't contain aluminum.The most common type of aluminum in antacids is aluminum hydroxide, which is transformed by hydrochloric acid in the stomach to aluminum chloride, which is easily absorbed in the intestines. Drinking citrus juice such as orange or grapefruit, or taking vitamin C within an hour or two of taking an antacid can greatly increase the absorption of aluminum.

Aluminum is also put into deodorants designed to be absorbed through the skin, creating daily source of aluminum consumption. Toothpaste is another source of aluminum compounds that can be avoided. Your local health food store will have aluminum-free deodorants and toothpastes.

Although aluminum pots and pans are not as large a source of aluminum as food additives, they remain

a daily source of aluminum consumption for those
who use them. Acidic foods such as tomatoes and coffee leach more aluminum from pots and pans, and
there is evidence that as they age they corrode, increasing levels of aluminum ingested. It's safer for
your health in the long run to use stainless steel pots
or pans with copper or aluminum outer bottoms to
conduct heat evenly, or you can use glass cookware.

ARSENIC

When I think of arsenic I think of Victorian-era detec-
tives on the trail of an arsenic poisoning, and indeed
for centuries it was one of the most popular ways to
kill someone else or commit suicide. Arsenic accumulates in the body, so taking very small amounts over a
long period of time will eventually cause poisoning.
It's interesting that among the "bad" trace minerals,
arsenic is not the most potently toxic. In fact the
"good" trace mineral fluoride is a much more potent
toxin than arsenic and was used as a rat poison before
it started being dumped into our municipal water supplies. (See page 21 for a more in-depth discussion of
water fluoridation.)

It may also surprise you to know that your body
needs arsenic—it is a necessary nutrient—although in
extremely small amounts, which you easily get just by
eating and drinking. In industrialized countries it's
much more likely that you're getting an overdose of
arsenic via industrial smokestacks, fungicides, pesticides,
herbicides and cigarette smoke.

Excess arsenic can cause high blood pressure; skin
abnormalities such as odd pigmentation, lesions and psoriasis; diarrhea; symptoms of heartburn and indigestion;
cancer; and poor circulation. There is also some evidence that chronic overexposure to arsenic can be a
causative factor in diabetes.

CADMIUM

Our major source of overexposure to the trace mineral cadmium is agricultural dependence on superphosphate fertilizers. Crops grown with them will absorb higher than normal levels of cadmium from the soil. Cadmium is not only toxic in and of itself in small amounts, it also displaces zinc, one of our most essential trace minerals. Cadimium replaces zinc in plants and animals, and is absorbed in greater amounts when zinc is deficient. Thus, like many of the toxic trace minerals, there is a double jeopardy, with overexposure to cadmium causing a deficiency of zinc and the potential for all the resulting illnesses. This is one of the best reasons I can think of to eat organic fruits and vegetables, aside from not being exposed to pesticides.

Cadmium is also an industrial waste product, and can be poisonous in doses as small as three parts per million. Alcoholic drinks like wine and whiskey are relatively high in cadmium, and cigarette smoke is a significant source. In fact, cadmium is probably one of the main sources of illness in those exposed to second-hand smoke. Pregnant women who smoke are more likely to give birth to zinc-deficient babies.

Cadmium also blocks the absorption of iron. In studies on the effects of cadium done with rodents, the immune system was compromised. Overexposure to cadmium also causes lung, kidney and liver disease, high blood pressure, and may play a role in Alzheimer's disease.

LEAD

According to the medical journal *Lancet*, some historians believe that lead contamination in wine decanters and other cookware in ancient Rome lead to its downfall, due to widespread lead poisoning among the upper classes. As farfetched as this theory might sound, it's not implausible, because the effects of lead poisoning are subtle and insidious, and lead to deterioration of the brain.

More recently, prior to the 1970s, lead was widely used in the U.S. in interior house paint. For this reason, lead is still an incredibly common source of poisoning, especially among children. If you live in one of the estimated 40 million houses in the U.S. that still has lead-based paint inside, you, your family and pets may be breathing lead-laden dust. It's more than worth it, if you live in a house built prior to 1976, to have your house dust- or paint-tested for lead.

If you do find that you have high levels of lead in your house paint or dust, it's important to cover it or remove it. If you remove it, be sure to take precautions not to breathe the dust created, or allow your family and pets to breathe it. Small children and pregnant women should not be allowed in a house where leaded paint is being removed. If you have lead paint on the outside of your house, it can wash off the side of the house and into the soil, polluting areas where children play or where pets spend time.

Those children most susceptible to lead poisoning live in urban slums where paint is peeling and there was, prior to the early 1990s when leaded gasoline was finally phased out, excessive lead in the air from car exhaust.

And here's the typical toxic trace mineral double jeopardy: zinc deficiency can exacerbate lead poisoning, and zinc supplementation may prevent it. While those in poverty in the U.S. aren't typically starving, their nutrition tends to be very poor, with an emphasis on refined white flours, chips, soda, sugary foods and other processed foods devoid of the essential trace minerals such as zinc. Children from low-income families have been shown to be deficient in dietary zinc, so not only are they over-exposed to lead, they are deficient in the very mineral that could help them avoid lead poisoning.

But lead doesn't just take up where zinc left off. Where lead is present in high levels, and calcium and magnesium are low, the body will take up lead instead of calcium and magnesium. Sufficient dietary calcium and magnesium can also help prevent lead poisoning.

Premature infants also tend to be deficient in zinc. Lead poisoning in children can cause mental retardation, stunted growth, hearing loss, anemia, high blood pressure, hyperactivity, aggressiveness, kidney disease, poor coordination, learning disabilities, and lower IQ. According to a report published in the *Journal of the American Medical Association,* a study that evaluated 503 first grade children for lead exposure found that higher levels of lead were associated with antisocial and delinquent behavior. When nutrition is very poor and lead exposure very high, even death may result.

Another source of lead is tap water polluted by old plumbing soldered with lead. The EPA (Environmental Protection Agency) estimates that one out of every six households in America have toxic levels of lead in their water. Tin cans soldered with lead used to be a source of lead poisoning in the U.S., and in many countries still are. Children may chew on toys with lead-based paints. Cigarette smoke is a source of lead. Lead crystal decanters, if used to store wine or other alcoholic or acidic beverages, can be a significant source of lead. Even a lead crystal glass filled with wine will leach tiny amounts of lead.

One of the most common sources of lead poisoning among adults in North America is ceramic pots, plates, cups, pitchers, casserole dishes and other cookware and food storage containers bought in foreign countries that don't regulate lead content, such as Mexico,

South America and Asia. If you buy these items outside of North America, I recommend you test them for lead before eating off them or using them to store food.

Symptoms of lead poisoning in adults can include confusion, headaches, constipation, fatigue, weight loss, high blood pressure, kidney disease, degenerative brain diseases, reproductive abnormalities and digestive problems. According to a study done at Harvard Medical School, even low levels of lead poisoning can cause kidney dysfunction in older men. Over-exposure to lead is also associated with cancer, probably because lead interferes with the production of glutathione, your body's first level of antioxidant defense.

MERCURY

The single biggest source of exposure to the toxic trace mineral mercury is dental fillings called amalgams, which contain a mix of metals, including mercury. Because mercury is a liquid metal at room temperature, and changes easily with changes in temperature and pressure, it readily gives off fumes which are inhaled by those with amalgam fillings.

Unfortunately, the toxicity of mercury fillings is not acknowledged by the American Dental Association, presumably due to fear of billions of dollars in class action lawsuits if they admit to the dangers of this extremely toxic and volatile heavy metal. In other countries mercury amalgams have been well studied, and it is clear that the more mercury amalgam fillings a person has, the higher the mercury concentrations in their blood and urine. Both dentists and dental assistants frequently show symptoms of mercury poisoning. Germany and Sweden have banned the use of mercury in dental fillings.

I strongly recommend that you not have any new

mercury amalgams put in, and if you are suffering from symptoms of mercury poisoning, have them taken out and replaced with porcelain fillings. (Gold fillings can contain high levels of cadmium.) There is no perfect substance to use for filling cavities in teeth, but porcelain seems to be the most benign right now.

Mercury is yet another heavy metal that is a common by-product of industrial wastes, and it is also a common waste product in hospitals. It is often dumped into waterways or the ocean, where it is ingested by shellfish and fish. Large fish that live near coastlines often have very high levels of mercury in their flesh. Swordfish and large tuna have the highest levels of mercury.

Mercury is one of the most toxic of the heavy metals, as it inhibits the body's use of the important B vitamin folic acid, and alters protein structures, which are involved in every aspect of bodily function.

Symptoms of mercury poisoning can include birth defects in the children of mothers exposed to it in utero, and central nervous system damage such as is seen in multiple sclerosis and Alzheimer's disease. Other symptoms include insomnia, anorexia, chronic fatigue, depression, headaches, diarrhea, irregular heartbeat, hair loss, irritability, kidney damage, loss of sex drive and muscle weakness. Mercury suppresses the immune system and creates a high susceptibility to infection.

If you break a thermometer in your home and spill mercury, cleaning it up can cause signficant amounts of mercury to escape into the air, carpets and dust of the house. Pregnant women and small children should be removed from the room for at least 24 hours, and the mercury should be carefully scooped up and placed in a closed glass container. The container should be disposed of at a hazardous waste facility. Then the area where the mercury spilled should be carefully vacuumed up, and the bag immediately disposed of.

NICKEL

Nickel is a trace mineral that is needed for the maintenance of health in very small amounts, but can quickly become toxic. Nickel is found in our RNA, and is thought to play a role in enzyme function. Overexposure to nickel can cause heart disease, cancer, skin disorders and thyroid malfunction. Since nickel is not a commonly used metal, overexposure to it is rare.

TIN

Poisoning from tin used to be a major health problem due to canning and storage of food in tin containers with no inner coating, but today it is rare. Caution should be used when eating canned foods outside North America. Some processed foods may contain tin-based preservatives and stabilizers.

Overexposure to tin may interfere with the body's production of glutathione, an important antioxidant, and block the absorption of copper, zinc and iron.

CHELATION THERAPY AND OTHER DETOXIFIERS

Mainstream medicine is largely at a loss to effectively handle heavy metal poisoning, but for years alternative doctors and other health-care professionals have sucessfully used chelation therapy to rid the body of these toxins and also to treat heart disease. Chelation therapy is controversial largely because it competes with prescription drugs and is a safe and effective alternative to them. Opponents claim that EDTA (ethylene diamine tetraacetic acid), the synthetic amino acid used in chelation, can produce kidney damage, but this is caused by factors such as dosage and biochemistry that are now taken into account, and there hasn't been an instance of kidney damage with EDTA use since the early 1960s.

Chelation therapy uses EDTA or other chelating agents, given intravenously over a period of many weeks or months in 20-30 treatments. At the same time, essential vitamins and minerals are given. EDTA essentially latches onto heavy metals that have accumulated in the tissues, combining with them to form compounds that can be excreted from the body. Chelation therapy is well studied, and has been used in at least half a million people. Remarkable results have been achieved using it for children with lead poisoning, and in adults with heart disease, Alzheimer's disease and arthritis.

Substances found in seaweed called alginates have been found to bind with some heavy metals, including strontium, cadmium, barium, radium and lead. Regularly adding dried seaweed products to meals can be a kind of health insurance against heavy metal poisoning.

Saunas and sweat baths are said to sweat out heavy metals, but this is hard on the body if you are already weakened by toxins.

One of the best allies against the accumulation of heavy metals in the body is proper nutrition. Getting plenty of the "good" trace minerals and enough of the body's other needed nutrients for optimal health will give your body the armament it needs to fight heavy metals.

GLOSSARY

absorption The process by which nutrients are passed into the bloodstream.

alkaline Containing an acid-neutralizing substance (being alkaline, sodium bicarbonate is used for excess acidity in foods).

amino acid chelates Chelated minerals that have been produced by many of the same processes nature uses to chelate minerals in the body; in the digestive tract, nature surrounds the elemental minerals with amino acid, permitting them to be absorbed into the bloodstream.

amino acids The organic compounds from which proteins are constructed; 22 amino acids have been identified as necessary to the human body; nine are known as essential—histidine, isoleucine, leucine, lysine, total S-containing amino acids, total aromatic amino acids, threonine, tryptophan, and valine—and must be obtained from food.

anorexia Abnormal fear of becoming obese, a persistent aversion to food, a distorted self-image, and severe loss of weight.

antioxidant A substance that can protect another substance from oxidation; added to foods to keep oxygen from changing the food's color.

arthritis Inflammation of joints.

arteriosclerosis A disease of the arteries characterized by hardening, thickening, and loss of elasticity of the arterial walls; results in impaired blood circulation.

assimilation The process whereby nutrients are used by the body and changed into living tissue.

asthma A condition of lungs characterized by a decrease in diameter of some air passages; a spasm of the bronchial tubes or swelling of their mucous membranes.

atherosclerosis A process whereby fatty deposits in the walls of arteries make the walls thick and hard, narrowing the arteries; a form of arteriosclerosis.

autoimmunity An abnormal condition whereby the body produces antibodies against its own tissues.

beta-carotene A plant pigment which can be converted into two forms of vitamin A.

carcinogen A cancer-causing substance.

cardiovascular Relating to the heart and blood vessels.

carotene An orange-yellow pigment occurring in many plants and capable of being converted into vitamin A in the body.

catalyst A substance that modifies, especially increases, the rate of chemical reaction without being consumed or changed in the process.

chelation A process by which mineral substances are changed into an easily digestible form.

cholesterol A white, crystalline substance, made up of various fats; naturally produced in vertebrate animals and humans; important as a precursor to steroid hormones and as a constituent of cell membranes.

coenzyme A substance that combines with other substances to form a complete enzyme; nonprotein and usually a B vitamin.

collagen The primary organic constituent of bone,

cartilage and connective tissue (becomes gelatin through boiling).

demineralization The loss of minerals or salts from bone and tissue.

diuretic Tending to increase the flow of urine from the body.

endocrine Producing secretions passed directly to the lymph or blood instead of into a duct; to do with the endocrine glands or the hormones they produce.

enzyme A protein substance found in living cells that brings about chemical changes; necessary for digestion of food; compounds with names ending in -ase.

FDA Food and Drug Administration.

gland An organ in the body where certain substances in the blood are separated and converted into secretions for use in the body (such as hormones) or to be discharged from the body (such as sweat); nonsecreting structures similar to glands, like lymph nodes, are also known as glands.

glucose Blood sugar; a product of the body's assimilation of carbohydrates and a major source of energy.

HDL High-density lipoprotein; HDL is sometimes called "good" cholesterol because it is the body's major carrier of cholesterol to the liver for excretion in the bile.

hemoglobin Molecule necessary for the transport of oxygen by red blood cells; iron is an essential component.

homeostasis The body's physiological equilibrium.

hormone A substance formed in endocrine organs and transported by body fluids to activate other specifically receptive organs, cells or tissues.

hydrochloric acid An acid secreted in the stomach; a main part of gastric juice.

immune Protected against disease.

insulin A hormone, secreted by the pancreas, that helps regulate the metabolism of sugar in the body.

LDL Low-density lipoprotein; sometimes referred to as "bad" cholesterol, LDLs easily become oxidized and carry cholesterol through the bloodstream; studies show high levels can increase risk of coronary artery disease (CAD).

metabolism The processes of physical and chemical change whereby food is synthesized into living matter until it is broken down into simpler substances or waste matter; energy is produced by these processes.

organic Describes any chemical containing carbon; or any food or supplement made with animal or vegetable fertilizers; or produced without synthetic fertilizers or pesticides and free from chemical injections or additives.

oxalates Organic chemicals found in certain foods, especially spinach, which can combine with calcium to form calcium oxalate, an insoluble chemical the body cannot use.

oxidation The way in which certain types of altered oxygen molecules cause biochemical reactions; examples are browning of apples and rancidity in oil.

protein A complex substance containing nitrogen which is essential to plant and animal cells; ingested proteins are changed to amino acids in the body.

RDA Recommended Dietary Allowances as established by the Food and Nutrition Board, National Academy of Sciences, National Research Council.

T-Cells White blood cells, manufactured in the thymus, which protect the body from bacteria, viruses, and cancer-causing agents, while controlling the production of B-cells which produce antibodies, and unwanted production of potentially harmful T-cells.

toxicity The quality or condition of being poisonous, harmful, or destructive.

toxin An organic poison produced in living or
dead organisms.

triglycerides Fatty substances in the blood.

USRDA United States Recommended Daily Allowances.

vitamin Any of about fifteen natural compounds essential in small amounts as catalysts for processes in
the body; most cannot be made by the body and
must come from diet.

BIBLIOGRAPHY

Bigazzi, Pierluigi E., "Autoimmunity and Heavy Metals," *Lupus*, 1994;3:449-453.

DiCyan, E., *A Beginner's Introduction to Trace Minerals*, Keats Publishing, New Canaan, Conn., 1984

Earth Matters, issue # 30, Friends of the Earth, London, Summer 1996.

Hauser, Robert, A., et al., "Blood Manganese Correlates with Brain Magnetic Resonance Imaging Changes in Patients with Liver Disease," *Canadian Journal of Neurological Science*, May 1996;23(2):95-98.

Hendler, S., *The Doctor's Vitamin and Mineral Encyclopedia*, Fireside, NY, 1991.

Hu, Howard, M.D., ScD., et al., "The Relationship of Bone and Blood Lead to Hypertension: The Normative Aging Study," *JAMA*, April 17, 1996;275-(15):1171-1176.

Jensen, B., et al., *Empty Harvest*, Avery Publishing Group Inc., Garden City Park, N.Y., 1990.

Kim, Rokho, M.D., Dr.P.H., et al., "A Longitudinal Study of Low-Level Lead Exposure and Impairment of Renal Function, The Normative Aging Study" *JAMA*, April 17, 1996;275(15):1177-1181.

Laino, Charlene, "City Air Pollution Linked to Male Infertility," *Medical Tribune*, November 9, 1995;14.

Martlew, G., *Electrolytes, the Spark of Life*, Nature's Publishing, Ltd., Murdock, Fla., 1994.

McClanahan, Mark, A., "Mercury Contamination in the Home," *The Lancet*, April 13, 1996;347:1044-1045.

Mesch, U., et al., "Lead Poisoning Masquerading as Chronic Fatigue Syndrome," *The Lancet*, April 27, 1996;347:1193.

Needleman, Herbert, L., et al., "Bone Lead Levels and Delinquent Behavior," *JAMA*, February 7, 1996;275(5):363-369.

Rader J.I., "Anti-nutritive Effects of Dietary Tin," *Adv. Exp. Med. Biol.*, 1991; 289:509-24.

Rahman, Mahfuzar and Axelson, Olav, "Diabetes Mellitus and Arsenic Exposure: A Second Look at Case-Control Data From a Swedish Copper Smelter," *Occupational and Environmental Medicine*, 1995;52:773-774.

Schmitt, Nicholas, "Could Zinc Help Protect Children From Lead Poisoning," *Canadian Medical Association Journal*, January 1, 1996;154(1):13-14.

Schroeder, H., *The Trace Elements and Man*, Devin-Adair, Greenwich, Conn., 1973

Sehnert, K.W., Clague, A.F. and Cheraskin, E., "Improvement in Renal Function Following EDTA Chelation and Multi-Vitamin-Trace Mineral Therapy: A Study in Creatinine Clearance," *Med. Hypotheses*, Nov 1984;15(3):301-4.

Somer, E., *The Essential Guide to Vitamins and Minerals*, HarperCollins, New York, 1995.

Stadtler, Von P., "Amalgam," *Occupation and Environment*, 1995;43:163-171.

Vaughn, L. et al., *Prevention Magazine's Complete Book of Vitamins and Minerals*," Wings Books, Avenel, N.J., 1994.

Dr. Earl Mindell's

What You Should Know About Homeopathic Remedies

INTRODUCTION

Homeopathy is a healing art that I am not an expert in, but since it is such an effective and safe part of natural healing, I'm including this basic guide to homeopathy in the "What You Should Know" series. Used according to its principles, homeopathy is a powerful tool for healing, especially when used in consultation with an experienced homeopath.

I consider this book a guide to nonserious conditions. If you have a condition such as diabetes, heart disease or severe arthritis, I strongly recommend that you work with an experienced homeopathic practitioner who can offer you the full benefit of these powerful remedies.

Some homeopathic remedies work very quickly and noticeably. For example, with some types of flu, the flu remedy Oscillococcinum can cure symptoms in a matter of hours. Arnica used promptly on a bruise can keep bruising symptoms to a minimum. But if it has taken you a long time to get an illness, a homeopathic remedy is most likely going to take some time, from a few weeks to a few months, to have its effect.

Like all truly effective forms of alternative medicine, homeopathy takes the whole person into account, including the physical, emotional, mental and spiritual levels. It is a form of medicine best used, most of the time, with attention to its principles and with awareness of all the detail that it is capable of addressing. As you delve into homeopathy, and learn to apply its remedies to yourself, you will learn more about an entirely new dimension of yourself, in fascinating detail. When you or your homeopath come upon the correct remedy, you will be amazed at how accurately the list of symptoms for that remedy fits your specific problem.

This guide was written with the assistance of homeopathic practitioner, teacher and author David Dancu, and I recommend that if you want to learn more about homeopathy you take advantage of his book, listed in the reference section in the back of this book, as well as the other works listed. And as I said above, I also recommend that when working with serious conditions, you work with a homeopathic practitioner who can give you the full advantage of the powerful homeopathic remedies.

CHAPTER 1

The History, Science and Philosophy of Homeopathy

Homeopathy originated in the 19th century as a result of the work of a German doctor, Samuel Hahnemann. It is founded on some very specific principles and an extensive list of tested remedies. The remedies are based on natural substances found to have various effects when taken in medicinal doses. The success of homeopathy as a safe and effective form of healing led to growth in its popularity and use throughout the century. As a practice, it was only overtaken when the developing science of modern medicine came to be favored by the medical establishments of North America and Europe.

Almost a century later, the drawbacks and dangers associated with conventional medicine have become obvious. Tranquilizer addiction, birth defects from pregnancy medications, and side effects of common medicines like aspirin, are a few examples of issues which have exposed a darker side to standard medical treatments. Many patients and doctors alike have been prompted to try approaches of a more consistently safe and compassionate nature such as homeopathy.

The tide has turned again in favor of the ancient tradition of medicine which sees the physician in service to the natural power of the body to heal itself. The trend in 20th-century medicine has been toward control and dominance of physical systems in isolation, treating symptoms and pain over and above underlying conditions and causes. Valuable knowledge and techniques have resulted, but often at great cost to the long term health of patients. The aim now is to combine modern developments with the understanding and usefulness of older, proven practices, including homeopathy.

THE LAW OF SIMILARS

Has anyone ever recommended that you "swallow a hair of the dog that bit you?" As a hangover cure it leaves a lot to be desired, but the idea of treating symptoms with a little of a substance that causes them is actually very sound. Known as the "Law of Similars," the theory is ancient. It was part of the writings of philosophers and physicians from Hippocrates to St. Augustine. Herbalists long ago applied a primitive version of the Law of Similars, in the form of the "The Doctrine of Signatures." Some plants were selected for medicinal use because they resembled in some way the part of the body to be treated. The speckled surface of a lungwort leaf, for instance, looks like a lung. Sure enough, modern science shows that the silica in lungwort restores elasticity to lungs and extracts of the plant are useful for reducing bronchial mucus.

A more refined concept of "similarity" was proposed in the 1790s by Samuel Hahnemann.

Unhappy with the increase of the barbaric medical practices of his time such as bloodletting, cupping and mercury poisoning, Hahnemann had quit his medical practice. When he turned to the translation of foreign medical and herbal publications, he began to question their theories and observations, and apply them to his own knowledge of healing.

Folk medicine from South America had produced a treatment for malaria, the world's number one killer disease of the 17th century. Powdered bark from the pretty cinchona tree proved a potent remedy. Known as quinine, cinchona extract is finding favor again today as malarial parasites have become resistant to synthetic drugs. In Hahnemann's time, herbalists believed cinchona's effectiveness was due to its bitterness. Hahnemann was not satisfied with this explanation, since many other bitter herbs were of no help.

Deciding to test the Law of Similars, he dosed himself with extract of cinchona bark. Remarkably, the healthy doctor was inflicted for a short time with symptoms very like those of malaria. This was the first of what Hahnemann called "provings." He continued with the help of colleagues, family and friends to conduct further tests on different substances, keeping detailed records of the results. The provings added further evidence that a cure of symptoms could result from taking herbs, minerals, elements or certain known toxins which actually induced similar responses in healthy people. To summarize his theory, Dr. Hahnemann coined the word "homeo-

pathy" from the Greek words "homoios" for similar and "pathos" for suffering.

HAHNEMANN'S ORGANON AND MATERIA
MEDICA

Hahnemann's first book on homeopathy, *The Organon of Rational Medical Science*, was published in
1810. The Organon set out the ideas and philosophy of homeopathy, and Hahnemann explained
his systematic approach and theories. These were
developed scientifically from the standpoint of
someone with a medical degree who was also an
authority on metal poisoning and toxicology.

The powerful effects observed by Hahnemann
in provings were achieved using highly diluted
amounts of the substances involved which, in a
few cases, were known poisons. The diluted
agents became homeopathic remedies. Over 400
of them were fully described, complete with provings, in his own materia medica, or medical
textbook.

Hahnemann's teachings spread slowly throughout Germany, meeting opposition from the entrenched medical establishment. His work was
regarded as a threat to much of the German
medical world, since he advocated small and limited doses which would not generate large pharmaceutical or practice profits. Personality played
a role, too, as Hahnemann's blunt, undiplomatic
style won him few friends in established circles.

In spite of the opposition, Hahnemann ex-
panded his writings, refining and adding remedies which led to four further editions of the
Organon during his lifetime. Through his work

with patients, he amassed an additional four volumes of information and cures compiled from cases and patient notes. A sixth *Organon* manuscript lay unpublished until it was found in 1920. This was more than 75 years after Hahnemann's death at age 88, in 1843, some time before homeopathy reached its 19th-century height. The changes and additions to homeopathic theory contained in the sixth *Organon* are major, yet not widely used by many modern homeopaths. The successful results achieved using the first five editions have created a reluctance to change.

THE PHILOSOPHY OF HOMEOPATHY

Even before publication of the *Organon*, Hahnemann's published writings demonstrated a refinement and philosophy that contrasted sharply with the crude thinking behind the common medical practices of the day. Unlike most physicians, he stressed the importance of exercise, diet and hygiene. He was aware of the pioneering work of contemporaries such as Edward Jenner on the smallpox vaccine, and was eager to advance the techniques of the ordinary physician.

Hahnemann's 1796 summary of three main approaches to medical treatment remains valid today. The first type of treatment could remove a known cause of a disease. A second form worked to oppose the effects of a disease, such as antacids to relieve heartburn, for example. The third, and superior type in his view, was treatment with similars designed to support the self-healing capabilities of the body. This was the essence of homeopathy. Hahnemann regarded homeopathic treatment, and prevention, as the only truly valid approaches to medicine. Each leads to the maintenance or active restoration of health rather than to the removal or suppression of disease factors.

Hahnemann understood the role of disease agents, but emphasized the idea that each person has a predisposition, or tendency, to get certain types of illness. He observed that agents act as triggers for disease, but not in all cases, and with worse consequences for some people than others. For example, the flu may afflict half the people in the office, and the other half may be unaffected. This led him to argue that the condition of the person is of greater importance than the disease agent. Included in this concept was the idea of the *vital force* of the individual, a term used by Hahnemann to explain the constant, automatic drive of an organism to stay in a healthy state.

HOMEOPATHY IN THE 19TH CENTURY

An increasing number of followers led to the rapid spread of homeopathy to almost all European countries as well as the United States, Mexico, Cuba and Russia. Eventually it would also reach South America and India. One of the main reasons for the growth in homeopathy was its superior effect in the treatment of epidemics such as typhoid fever and cholera which swept over Europe and America in the last century. When yellow fever hit the southern states of America in 1878, death rates were one third fewer in patients treated with homeopathy than in those receiving orthodox treatment. In London, in 1854, over half the cholera patients in conventional hospitals died, in contrast to just over 16 percent in homeopathic hospitals.

Homeopathy was introduced to the United States in 1825. Demand for homeopathy in America stemmed initially from German communities. Philadelphia saw the establishment of the first homeopathic medical school in 1833. The school was founded by Dr. Constantine Hering who had originally taken up the cause against Hahnemann in Germany. Aimed at disproving the discoveries of homeopathy, Hering's research did the opposite! Convinced by a natural form of healing free of side effects, the former enemy became a dedicated ally. Hering went on to write many books on homeopathy and himself worked as a homeopathic practitioner.

Another famous American homeopath was James Kent, M.D. who was based in Philadelphia from the early 1890s. Many years of work, involving the treatment of over 30,000 patients, and lectures and notes from other materia medica, led to the publication in 1897 of *Kent's Repertory*. As a comprehensive listing of symptoms and remedies, this source is still used by homeopaths everywhere.

Leading proponents such as Hering and Kent worked to meet the rising call for homeopathy in America which, by the 1880s, had created 100 hospitals and 20 medical colleges. Homeopathy was taught at Boston, Iowa, Michigan and Minnesota universities. At that time, twenty percent of physicians were homeopaths. The gentle approach of homeopathy, free of side effects, and caring for the patient as a whole, was in contrast to the rising use of synthetic drugs and treatment only of symptoms in standard American medical practice.

PRESSURES AGAINST HOMEOPATHY

Patients in the 18th century were accustomed to brutal techniques like mercury dosing, which frequently caused teeth to fall out, and bloodletting often "until four fifths of the blood contained in the body are drawn away!" Homeopathy provided an attractive alternative. Ordinary folk and the elite of society, including politicians and the wealthy, patronized homeopaths, competing with standard physicians. The resulting jealousy and fear meant homeopathy became the target of official repression. The founding of the American Institute of Homeopathy in 1844 was followed, as a direct response, two years later by the formation of the American Medical Association (AMA). Doctors with any connections to homeopathic practices were barred from the AMA. Members of the AMA were not even permitted to consult homeopaths.

The pharmaceutical industry also perceived itself threatened by homeopathy. Scientists in the 18th century had discovered that the active chemicals of medicinal plants could be isolated. During the 19th century, chemists focused on the extraction and synthesis of these potent substances. In the minds of industry and public alike was the idea of quick-fix, one-stop medicine. Long term effects and treatment of underlying conditions came to be largely ignored. New, synthesized drugs were often speedily effective against urgent symptoms. Side effects went unidentified as drugs could treat those, too, masking true medicinal changes in the body.

Additional pressure came when the United States government commissioned the Flexner Report in 1910. The intention was to assess medical education and to set standard practices. However, this was in the context of the rise of a limited chemical approach fixated on physical symptoms. The report led to the closure of many medical schools, including those teaching homeopathy. Homeopathy fell outside the narrow biochemical framework accepted and promoted by the medical establishment. It has to be added that homeopaths created their own vulnerability to attack. As a developing system, it accommodated proponents of different views on high and low dilutions and did not offer a consistent front to those attempting to undermine the subject. Millions of dollars' worth of grants were denied to homeopathic medical schools, and homeopathic hospitals became standard medical institutions.

Adding to the decline of homeopathy in the United Sates was a major lifestyle shift from slow-paced and rural to urban and mobile. Society no longer provided an easy fit for the typical family doctor who often treated the same patients for their entire lives. Finally, the advent of so-called "wonder drugs" in the 1940s saw homeopathy retreat outside the margins of medical practice.

HOMEOPATHY TODAY

It wasn't until the early 1970s that dissatisfaction within the medical field led to a revival of homeo-

pathy. Recognizing the ineffectiveness and often
downright harm of modern drugs, some physicians arranged to study in Greece where homeopathy was more widely practiced. Greek instructors
came to America to lecture on Hahnemann's
work, and so began the increase in popularity of
homeopathy seen in the United States today.

More than one-third of the U.S. population
now uses alternative remedies, including homeopathy. Complications from prescription drugs
result in 40 percent of hospitalizations and cause
20,000 to 30,000 deaths every year in the United
States. The comparative effectiveness and safety
of homeopathic remedies is being demonstrated
by more and more top-notch scientific studies
done by respected institutes. Studies done in
America, England, Germany, Holland and France
include research into homeopathic remedies for
cold and flu, skin ailments, allergies, insect bites
and stings, menopause and sports injuries.

In America, homeopathic remedies are now
recognized as medicines. They are freely available
in health and drug stores and come under the
jurisdiction of the Food and Drug Administration
(FDA). Some homeopathic remedies, such as ni-
troglycerine for certain heart ailments, have been
taken up by allopathic medicine and used in medicinal doses.

The Queen of England and Mother Theresa
have homeopathy in common! The Queen is at-
tended by a homeopathic physician and homeopathic remedies are used in Mother Theresa's
Calcutta hospital. Homeopathic medicines are
used in the practices of a fifth of German physicians and just under a third of French physicians.

In 1980, there were nearly 800 homeopathic doctors in France and around 200 in Britain. India boasts about 124 homeopathic medical schools and there is a sprinkling of schools and colleges in South America. About 450 homeopathic physicians practice in Argentina alone.

Aside from entrenched medical practice steered to a large degree by drug company interests, there has remained a mainstream reluctance to accept homeopathy. This has been due in part to the fact that no complete understanding of what makes homeopathy effective exists. Another factor is the lack of interest on the part of homeopaths to finding classifiable, physical causes to the symptoms it cures. Allopathic medicine has yet to move on to the position that the agents of disease are less important than the paths that lead to recovery and cure.

Those practicing homeopathy have begun to realize the need to move on as well, and accept the need for testing that meets the criteria of Western medicine as well as established techniques of proving. Perhaps the time has come for the gentle, proven techniques of homeopathy to gain acceptance alongside the best and safest of current established medical practices.

PUTTING HOMEOPATHY TO THE TEST

Homeopathy is an ongoing subject of research and an interesting one because the way it works is not completely understood, although there are some very convincing theories. Impartial and well executed studies include work on a range of subjects. In an article in the *British Medical Journal,*

107 controlled trials in homeopathy were reviewed by authors who were not themselves homeopaths. Most of the trials did not meet Western medicine protocals, but nevertheless, the authors were amazed at the amount of positive evidence that could still be gleaned. Many more trials are needed to satisfy scientific criteria, but headway is already being made.

Examples of recent homeopathic trials include a Harvard clinical study on Similasan Eye Drops # 2, an ophthalmic (eye) allergy medication containing extracts of honey bee, eyebright and cevadilla. Using a well-established test known as the Antigen Challenge, the drops were found to significantly reduce hay fever symptoms such as itching and bloodshot eyes.

According to a study published in the *The Lancet*, a homeopathic remedy was more effective than a placebo in relieving allergy symptoms (mainly due to dust mites) in 28 patients who also continued their conventional care. Patients taking the homeopathic remedy reported 33 percent fewer asthma symptoms, sustained for up to four weeks after the trial. Improvements were seen within one week from the start of the treatment. These results correlated with a 53 percent increase in histamine resistance for the treated group, while the placebo group saw a 7 percent decrease.

In a study of 81 children in Nicaragua, reported in the journal *Pediatrics*, children treated with a homeopathic medicine for diarrhea recovered more quickly than those given a placebo.

A 1995 clinical study of 68 volunteers, published in the *European Journal of Clinical Pharmacol-*

ogy, found a homeopathic gel to be significantly superior to a placebo in the treatment of mosquito bites.

Results such as these give a hint of the wide-ranging use and effectiveness of homeopathic medicines. It should be noted, too, that this is without the application of full homeopathic techniques, which require exact tailoring of remedies to the individual affected, not just the physical symptoms in isolation.

THE PRINCIPLES OF HOMEOPATHY

A basic, guiding principle of homeopathy was stated by Hahnemann in his *Organon*: "The highest ideal of therapy is to restore health rapidly, gently, permanently; to remove and destroy the whole disease in the shortest, surest, least harmful way, according to clearly comprehensible principles."

Hahnemann developed just such specific principles which are still followed, shaping the practice of all homeopaths today.

The Principle of The Like Remedy

A homeopathic remedy always follows the Law of Similars, as it is chosen for its ability to produce symptoms that are most like those of the person to be treated. For instance, the syrup of ipecacuanha will cause vomiting when ingested in its natural form. When diluted and potentized in the homeopathic form (this concept will be explained shortly), it prevents or eliminates vomiting and nausea. This is considered the foundation for homeopathic principles; whatever causes a specific reaction in an individual also cures that disharmony when taken in homeopathic dilution.

In homeopathy, symptoms are investigated in depth, covering physical signs, the nature of the illness, underlying level of health and energy, personality, trauma and inherited tendencies. The aim is always to look at the person as a whole. Remedies are chosen from a range that has been scientifically tested on healthy human beings to determine what symptoms they produce. The resulting list of symptoms is known as a remedy's "drug picture." One of the fundamental discoveries of homeopathy showed that the most effective remedy is the one whose drug picture most closely matches the individual's symptoms, or "clinical picture."

The Single Drug Principle

Many combination homeopathic remedies are effective for acute illnesses or conditions. In our fast-paced lives, when there isn't time to stop and review symptoms in depth, a combination remedy often does the trick. However, it will leave you without knowledge as to which homeopathic substance in particular was most effective. Combinations are not original homeopathic remedies, but derive more from the herbalist approach, where long tradition shows that different agents can enhance the effect of others.

Classic homeopathy calls for one remedy to be tried at a time so that its effects can be clearly seen. If unrelated symptoms or symptoms not ex-

perienced before should occur after taking a homeopathic dose, the remedy should be
discontinued. Any ill effects, however, will be
short lived.

The Principle of the Small Dose and Potentization

One fascinating discovery made by Hahnemann
was that the effectiveness of a homeopathic remedy increased the more the dose was diluted.
Hahnemann observed that when a match was
achieved between symptoms and a remedy, the
patient would be very sensitive to the remedy. A
much lower dose was needed for a positive reaction than in a case without a good symptom
match or in a healthy person. This spurred Hahnemann to continue lowering dilutions to find
curative doses as well as to eradicate toxicity.

Part of the process of dilution involved vigorous
shaking, called succussion, to achieve useable, ho-
mogeneous chemical solutions. Hahnemann later
named this process *potentization* or *dynamization.*
Achieving increased potency with lower doses is
in contrast to allopathy, where normally the dose
is *increased* to produce more effect.

In his fifth edition of the *Organon*, Hahnemann
sets out a range of potencies. The most commonly used dilutions are given in centesimal and
decimal amounts. In centesimal potencies, one
drop of the active substance is dissolved in 99
drops of distilled water, alcohol or glycerine. Substances which cannot be dissolved in this way are
ground up with lactose (milk sugar). A resulting
solution is called the mother tincture, which is
then used as the basis for further dilution, pro-

ducing potency ranges termed 1c right up to 100,000c or cm. Decimal, or x potencies, involve dilution of the mother tincture in just 9 drops of water or alcohol. X potencies range from 1x to 200x. Much weaker solutions, known as lm potencies, were recommended by Hahnemann in his sixth *Organon*, but these have not been widely used.

The Principle of the Infrequent Dose

Homeopathic remedies are only administered as necessary. With acute, self-limiting conditions such as bruises and colds, the right remedy can produce changes four to eight hours or even sooner after the first dose. Patience, however, is part of the key to homeopathic treatment of more serious conditions. Days and sometimes weeks are allowed for effects to be seen and doses are not repeated when improvement is maintained. There is no expectation of the long, continuous courses of medicine often seen with allopathic medicine.

The Principle of Noninterference with the Body's Natural Response

This principle recognizes the body's innate ability to heal itself. There is much greater knowledge today than during Hahnemann's time of the numerous repair functions of the body. When struck by illness or injury, the body automatically triggers healing processes on many levels. For example, fevers burn off infections, endorphins flow as natural pain killers, and white blood cells destroy foreign agents. Although the exact nature of the healing systems was not known to Hahnemann, he recognized and summarized these kinds of responses and their regulatory mechanism as vital reactions.

We now know exactly how conventional 19th century medical practices such as bloodletting would have literally drained the body's ability to respond to infection. Hahnemann observed as much, even though he was unaware of the precise processes being crudely ignored. For this reason he formulated the principle of noninterference. Homeopathy is designed to support the healing functions of the body, shortening the time needed to restore health.

The Principle of Treatment of the Whole Person

Hahnemann observed that the body's ability to fight disease and repair itself was directed by what he referred to as the *vital force*. This was his description of the capacity of organisms to self-regulate always in the direction of survival and therefore health. Even today, this function is not well understood, but, like Hahnemann, we see it affected by moods and emotions. Today, we can measure how immune cell numbers drop with depression or how our body's natural anticancer agents increase with happiness. By acknowledging a vital force, Hahnemann was addressing the large role played by the emotional, mental and spiritual levels of a person's health.

A good homeopathic assessment reviews a person's vitality and emotional state. If someone has a cold but still feels energetic, a more potent remedy will be tolerated. Similarly, acute symptoms such as a cold are not treated homeopathically without regard also to chronic conditions such as arthritis or indigestion.

Thorough training in all aspects of homeopathy leads to the most comprehensive and effective treatments. This is why it makes good sense to select a trained, experienced homeopath.

HOW DOES HOMEOPATHY WORK?

The answer to this question is not fully known. The powerful effect of the very diluted remedies used in homeopathy is a puzzling subject for researchers. Many dilutions are so high that no molecular trace of the original substance can be found. Homeopaths believe that the vigorous shaking at each level of dilution leaves the energy of the original dissolved substance imprinted on the medium of solution, something like an energetic blueprint, or fingerprint.

Various theories about the mechanisms of homeopathy are being tested. For example, electromagnetism may play a role, as it has been found that allergic manifestations occur in highly sensitive subjects contacting water treated with electromagnetic frequencies. Some investigations suggest that when pure water is treated with electromagnetic waves it gains new physical and chemical properties that are conserved for some time. It's true to say that the properties of water are in many ways still a mystery. Results of future work investigating homeopathic dilutions may yield interesting discoveries.

Homeopathy can be seen as influencing the energy fields of the body. Each human body is a unique pattern of energy flows and each cell has an electromagnetic or "bioelectric" field. A cell is an energy generator, functioning in harmony with every other cell to create an overall level of health. At times of illness, there are disharmonies in energy production and flows in the body.

It is thought that the properties of a correct homeopathic remedy for an ailment in some way resonate with and strengthen the body's efforts to realign its unbalanced energy flows.

WORKING WITH, NOT AGAINST, SYMPTOMS

When you take a dose of, say, antibiotics, the aim is to kill the organisms that have caused the symptoms of an infection. You might also take other drugs to bring down a fever or kill pain. This, of course, is very different from the approach taken by homeopathy. Allopathic treatment has a vital role in emergency treatment and it gets results because it often removes the source of an infection or condition. However, it usually does so with a blast of powerful substances that override the body's own defense mechanisms. In many cases, allopathic medicine simply suppresses symptoms and does not tackle root causes. This is true, for instance, of drugs for heartburn, sinus troubles and high blood pressure. In addition, the medicinal substances themselves frequently cause unwanted side effects which not uncommonly lead to the administration of yet more drugs.

In homeopathy, symptoms are regarded as outward signs of the body's efforts to repair itself. By taking tiny amounts of a substance which pro-

duces similar symptoms, a cure results because
the defense work of the body has been stimulated
and reinforced. In allopathic medicine, the disease often becomes harder to treat, as with bacteria that become resistant to antibiotics. The aim
of homeopathy is not to bypass the body's own
systems, but to support them. In this way the
body gains in its ability to fend off disease.

Release of Suppressed Symptoms

Hahnemann's provings showed that a remedy
can provoke an "occasional initial aggravation,"
the release of symptoms which have become suppressed. When a release is seen it is sometimes
referred to as a healing crisis. A release involves
the recurrence of old symptoms, usually for just
a few hours a day, but sometimes longer if they
were originally severe. A trained homeopathic
doctor will decide whether to prescribe a different remedy, reduce the potency, or wait out the
crisis.

In allopathic medicine, it is unlikely that a patient would be asked to consider past symptoms.
A reappearance of old symptoms may be seen as
incidental and/or subject to new treatment, or
mistaken as a sign that a successful treatment
should be changed. Allopathic medicine is unlikely to consider a recurrence of old symptoms
as a sign of recovery.

Disease as a Dynamic Condition

The tendency in allopathic medicine is to fit the
patient to a known disease. A doctor attempts to
pin down symptoms to a generally classified pat-

tern, in which the overall match is more important than any variations shown by an individual.
This is what medical doctors are taught in medical school: first they learn how to diagnose a disease, and then they learn which drug to prescribe
to treat the disease. We've all seen doctors prescribe a first choice of antibiotics and then a second, even a third, when the first was ineffective.
People have become used to being treated in
such a general fashion, since modern medicine
has established certain "molds" for illness to fit
into. At the same time, we accept that people
experience disease differently, recovering at different rates, responding to viruses with different
symptoms, requiring more or less rest. Yet despite
these observed differences, we've learned to accept nonindividualized treatment.

Homeopathy and the Holistic Approach

Holistic treatment does not single out one physical aspect or body part for treatment. It is an
approach that takes the whole person into account, rather than just physical symptoms. As an
holistic practice, homeopathy does not place the
disease in a compartment separate from the individual. Symptoms are seen to reflect ongoing, dy-
namic efforts by the body to return to a healthy
state, not as unwanted manifestations to be classified and stamped out in isolation from other
bodily functions.

In this way, homeopathy recognizes the inter-
dependency of all parts of the body. It also incor-
porates the role played by personality types so

that homeopathic treatments are tuned to each individual patient.

THE HOMEOPATHIC PHYSICIAN

Most physicians are well-intentioned and sincere in their vocation. The training of an allopathic doctor, however, is steered toward acceptance of a prescription drug culture, in which the medical world is greatly influenced by the pharmaceutical industry. The homeopath takes a more independent view, although his or her training in medical matters will be just as thorough. A homeopath perceives his or her prescriptions as supplementary rather than superior to the body's own powers. In practicing homeopathy, a physician will usually pay greater attention to the patient's general condition than an allopathic doctor. A desire to know a great deal about individual patients and their symptoms in great detail leads to much more time spent with them than is the norm in conventional medicine. Whereas a standard physician may see about 30 patients a day, spending about 10 minutes with each, a homeopathic doctor typically sees 8 to10 patients a day and spends about an hour with each one.

Like any other doctor, a homeopathic physician receives an M.D. degree and his or her state license to practice medicine. To qualify to practice homeopathy, he or she then goes on to a postgraduate course in the subject, followed by a period of work with a practicing homeopathic physician. Only a few states license homeopathic practitioners. Recommendations from others and experience count equally for conventional and homeopathic doctors.

What to Expect from a Homeopathic Physician

You may understand how a homeopathic doctor is different from an allopathic physician, but how does this affect treatment? Homeopathy sets out certain procedures as standard. As a result, patients can expect a basic similarity in the work of different homeopaths. As with doctors of all kinds, of course, each physician has his or her own style and character which will influence the way he or she practices.

One of the major preferences expressed by those who choose a homeopathic doctor is over the amount of time the physician is willing to spend with patients. An initial hour-long interview is typical, and feedback from patients is welcome in regard to the changes seen after taking a remedy. Important and specific use is made of patient-doctor time.

A standard element of homeopathy is the collection of information about the patient. This is known as "taking the case." From the first encounter with the patient, a homeopathic doctor is taking note of his or her condition. Factual information is recorded, including age, occupation, marital status and the patient's reason for visiting. A homeopath goes on from there to consider factors such as posture, complexion, stress level, and emotions as valuable clues to an individual's state of health. Considerable skill is needed for a homeopath to be sure of noting underlying traits, not just accept a doctor's-visit façade!

An interview notes not just physical symptoms, their onset, type and timing, but also personal history, which provides information about a patient's emotional and mental tendencies—if they are ambitious, inhibited or extroverted, for example. A history of family illness is also covered, to give an indication of any possible inherited conditions, and the individual's probable underlying physical strengths and weaknesses.

Symptoms are discussed in detail, determining how they have changed and if they vary over the day. In addition, the patient is asked to describe how his or her condition affects him or her, and if it has changed the way they react to their environment. Food preferences are important here, noting, for instance, if something is disliked that was previously favored.

The result of the initial interview is a comprehensive picture of the patient's state of health, specific symptoms, and personal response to their condition. The homeopathic physician uses the interview notes as the basis for prescribing a remedy without the need arising to first classify the illness.

Visiting a physician for a full homeopathic review results in the prescription of a single remedy. This is to avoid stimulating multiple responses in the body which cannot be definitely associated with a specific remedy. In other words, a homeopath's initial intention is to find only the remedy which is key to the illness. This approach is very different from an individual's educated purchase of a combination remedy for self-treatment.

Someone finding quick relief, say, from hay fever, isn't going to mind exactly which substance in a combination remedy produces the result. More severe conditions, however, merit a comprehensive investigation, which leads in traditional homeopathy to one remedy alone.

Diagnosis Comes Second to Symptoms

The pattern of symptoms observed by a homeopathic physician is used to point to a specific remedy rather than to a particular disease. This is called "constitutional prescribing," or matching the treatment to the person as a whole, not just the condition. Homeopaths do provide a diagnosis if one is needed, say, for insurance purposes, but the diagnosis is not used to provide the framework for action.

Out of perhaps a dozen main symptoms, the physician will usually judge five or so to be the strongest. One symptom may point to several remedies. Exactly which remedy is used is determined in cross-reference with the remedies suggested by the other leading symptoms. Usually, one remedy will match most of the symptoms. The physician checks the description of patient and symptoms listed under the remedy to insure it is indeed a clear match with the individual being treated. A good match between the "drug picture" and the "clinical picture" is confirmation that the right remedy has been selected. The remedy is prescribed and any dietary factors, such as coffee, which could interfere with its actions, are ruled out. Most homeopaths provide general advice about diet and lifestyle, since prevention of disease is a high priority in the homeopathic world. The first visit, however, is usually reserved for "taking the case" and dealing with immediate discomfort.

AGGRAVATION AS A COMMON RESPONSE

The old adage "you'll feel worse before you feel better" often holds truth in homeopathy. A patient is usually very sensitive to the right remedy, which produces symptoms most similar to his own. The right remedy will often provoke the defensive measures of the body, and often actually increases the intensity of symptoms for as long as a day or two. This syndrome of aggravation can also be the release of earlier, repressed symptoms.

An expert homeopath will be sure to confirm that any increase in symptoms is either a temporary, bearable worsening of symptoms or a renewal of old ones, rather than a new set of responses which are not connected to the original condition being treated.

KEEPING COSTS DOWN

One bonus of homeopathic treatment is that it is less costly than allopathic medicine. Visits are made less frequently and fewer diagnostic tests are ordered. A century and a half of research, provings and contributions to materia medica means that homeopathic pharmaceutical companies do not have to bear the huge costs of research and development of new drugs. A homeopathic physician prescribes from an established range of about 500 classically proven homeopathic substances, and a total of about 2,800 substances, which are produced without expensive hype and promotion. The result is medications for prescription and self-treatment which are cheaper than the conventional medicines. An allopathic doctor, in contrast, has a prescription list of about 10,000 available drugs whose high cost reflects the high price of their manufacture and promotion.

Homeopathic drugs are safe. The long history of their production and use has insured they are nontoxic. Modern medical drugs, on the other hand, lead to an estimated five to 10 million serious reactions every year. The costs of treating adverse drug reactions does not arise with homeopathy.

THE PATIENT'S ROLE

Anyone seeking homeopathic treatment benefits from a willingness to be honest and thorough in communication with the physician. A homeopathic patient-doctor relationship is a close and active one. The patient is not a passive recipient of advice and treatment. Finding an effective homeopathic remedy relies on good communication from a patient willing to convey a lot of information about his condition. With a remedy in use, the patient's job is to provide feedback about any and all changes. Strong communication creates a close and effective relationship between homeopathic patient and doctor. This helps the doctor ensure the appropriate medicine is in use and that no condition needing allopathic intervention has been missed. Unlike allopathic patients, who are expected to quietly and passively do as they are told without question, homeopathic patients are expected to speak up loud and clear!

CHAPTER 2

Self-Treating and Using Combination Remedies and Formulas

Combination remedies have been used in homeopathy since its beginnings. One of Samuel Hahnemann's first combinations, Causticum, was a mixture of slaked lime with a solution of potassium sulphate. Its effectiveness was clear and powerful. This unique combination remedy covers many conditions, including joint problems, emotional disharmonies, allergies, fibromyalgia, sinus problems, back pains, and multiple sclerosis.

There are several things to consider when choosing either a combination remedy or a combination of remedies. Most classical homeopaths use only single remedies, simply because they can determine the effect of that remedy without interaction of other forces. With each single remedy, there is a clear proving of what that remedy can cause.

Simplicity is the underlying key for using homeopathy, and single remedies provide the basis for maintaining that simplicity. Combinations, on the other hand, are easy to use for self-treatment, but may not be as effective for chronic conditions, such as asthma, arthritis, depression, anxiety or most other long-term illnesses.

Let's say I have been getting headaches frequently. They usually occur after stress or possibly from a reaction to car exhaust. There are three approaches to consider. The obvious and easy one is the traditional western philosophy of taking an aspirin to eliminate the headache. The second approach is to try a homeopathic combination containing five or six remedies, all generally specific for headaches, such as Nux Vomica, Spigilia, Sanguinaria or Lycopodium. One of these will probably work just fine, much like an aspirin.

The third approach, which is a more classical homeopathic approach, uses a different perspective, as it considers the cause of the headache, not just the symptom. One remedy is given based on the whole picture, rarely just the headache alone. This way, a determination is made on both the effect and the result, while also considering whether or not there were reactions in other parts of the body.

The first two approaches look to the symptom without consideration for the person or the cause. And there are obvious times when this approach is not only effective but necessary. Whenever possible though, a review of all symptoms will help to establish a deeper, more permanent healing.

In addition to having specific labels for various ailments, ranging from colds to asthma, combination remedies list a series of ingredients. Reputable companies make these combinations, based on sound homeopathic principles. They combine remedies which work for the ailment described on the label, specifically derived from established materia medica (a book describing remedies) and provings.

Each homeopathic remedy chosen is based on clear symptoms of mental, emotional and physical aspects. A good example is a remedy called pulsatilla. Emotionally, the symptom picture of this remedy is generally a codependent, weepy, timid, depressed, capricious and soft woman. Physically, she often has PMS, stomach or digestive disorders, hay fever, headaches, joint problems and is rarely thirsty, despite a dry mouth.

Typically she is also warm-blooded, with most of her symptoms being much worse either in the sun or in a stuffy, warm room. Her skin is frequently fair, she has light-colored hair and is overweight. Visualize a vine, clinging to the side of a building, and you have a good picture of Pulsatilla tendencies. A healthy person taking this remedy may exhibit some of the above symptoms. But this also demonstrates what it can cure when taken by someone who has similar' symptoms.

Every proven homeopathic remedy has its own unique portrait, some in more depth than others. And some are more specific to certain ailments, such as berberis for kidney and bladder problems. The number of proven remedies is about 2,800, with more added on a regular basis.

There are also quite a few substances being called homeopathic that have never been proven and have no relationship to cure other than the fact that they have been diluted. It takes time and effort to weed out the proven from the unproven, but the time taken may prevent ill effects or an unwanted proving on yourself.

All proven remedies are listed in a book called a materia medica. It gives necessary information and effects of each specific remedy. Ask your health food store to carry an inexpensive version for review purposes. You can also use this book and the others recommended in the back of the book for proven recommendations.

Remedies that are proven combinations often naturally occur that way. This list includes calcium and phosphorus, iron and phosphorus, sodium and sulphur and hundreds of others. The idea is to understand what the combination may create and what effect it will have on the body, once created.

For an acute problem or an emergency, combinations can be very helpful and effective. In chronic or long-term disharmonies, the combination remedies act much in the same way as an aspirin does, rarely getting to the cause, just giving temporary relief. And continued repetition is necessary to maintain that relief.

The following is a review of specific remedies in relation to general areas of the body. When considering a combination for a certain ailment, one or more of these remedies would generally be included. Keep in mind that each remedy may be valuable for more than one type of illness or ailment. For instance, Arsenicum Album is a single remedy used for allergies, sneezing, diarrhea, colitis, skin problems, respiratory ailments, shingles, headaches, food poisoning, fears, anxieties, compulsive disorders and depression. But it is best used when there is restlessness in conjunction with one of the above ailments, because otherwise it may not be as effective or long lasting.

The headings described below, along with related remedies, should be used as guidelines, rather than absolutes. Remember that some substances being called homeopathic remedies have never been proven, and unless one of the listed remedies is included, use caution in your selections.

The Head (including headache, injury, pains and congestion): Arnica; Aconite; Belladonna; China; Gelsemium; Glonine; Iris; Kali Bichromium; Lachesis; Natrum Muriaticum; Nux Vomica; Phosphorus; Pulsatilla; Sepia; Silica; Sulphur.

The Nose (including sinus, pains, congestion and discharges): Aconite; Allium Cepa; Arsenicum Iodatum; Belladonna; Calcarea Carbonica; Euphrasia; Hepar; Kali Bichromium; Lycopodium; Mercurius; Natrum Muriaticum; Pulsatilla; Silica; Sticta; Thuja.

The Mouth (including abscesses, odor, pains and infections): Arsenicum Album; Calcarea Carbonica and Phosphoricum; Camphora; China; Carbo Vegetabilisatablis; Hepar; Mercurius; Nitricum Acidum; Lachesis; Nux Vomica; Silica; Sulphur.

The Eyes (including injuries, vision, eruptions, discharges, inflammations, pains and styes): Apis; Aconite; Euphrasia; Ruta; Staphysagria; Causticum; Phosphorus; Pulsatilla; Natrum Muriaticum; Nitricum Acidum; Mercurius; Kreosotum; Rhus Tox; Silica.

The Ears (including infections, hearing, pains and tinnitus): Aconite; Belladonna; Chamomilla; Pulsatilla; Silica; Hepar Sulphuricum; Mercurius; Kali Bichromium; Sulphur; Causticum; Petroleum; Lycopodium; Sarsaparilla; China.

The Throat (including infection, inflammation and pains): Aconite; Apis; Arsenicum Album; Belladonna; Cantharis; Phytolacca; Sulphur; Phosphorus; Pulsatilla; Lycopodium; Mercurius; Lachesis; Natrum Muriaticum; Rhus Tox; Silica; Capsicum.

The Lungs (including inflammations, infections, breathing, coughs and discharges): Arsenicum Album; Antimonium Tart; Argentum Nitricum; Bryonia; Carcinosin; Drosera; Hepar; Kali Bichromium; Lachesis; Phosphorus; Rumex Tuberculinum; Spongia; Sambucus; Sulphur.

The Stomach (including digestion, gas, bloating, pains, cramps, appetite, hiccoughs and nausea): Antimonium Crudum; Argentum Nitricum; Arsenicum Album; Carbo Vegetabilisatablis; Calcarea Carbonica; China; Chelidonium; Ipecacuanha; Cocculus Indicus; Lachesis; Lycopodium; Nux Vomica; Aloe; Natrum Muriaticum; Pulsatilla.

Extremities (including joints, pains, bones, bruises, breaks, arthritis, inflammations, ligaments and strains): Arnica; Calcarea Carbonica; Calcarea Fluorica; Calcarea Phosphorica; Causticum; Colchicum; Cuprum; Silica; Symphytum;

Phosphorus; Plumbum; Bryonia; Rhus Tox Ruta; Ledum.

Female (including PMS, hormonal problems, cysts, herpes, pains, menopause, discharges and headaches): Belladonna; Calcarea Carbonica; Caulophyllum; Cimicifuga; Cyclamen; Ignacia; Lilium Tig; Natrum Muriaticum; Natrum Carbonicum; Natrum Phosphoricum; Phosphorus; Sepia; Pulsatilla; Platina; Sabina; Lycopodium; Thuja; Silica; Kreosotum; Medorrhinum; Nitricum Acidum.

Male (including herpes, impotence, erectile difficulty, prostate, pains, desires, infections and inflammations): Arsenicum Album; Argentum Nitricum; Calcarea Carbonica; Calcarea Sulphuricum; Causticum; Conium; Lycopodium; Nux Vomica; Medorrhinum; Lachesis; Thuja; Sabal; Sulphur; Mercurius.

Sleep (including insomnia, thoughts, disturbed, restless, anxious; too short or too long and unrefreshing): Arsenicum Album; Argentum Nitricum; Belladonna; Calcarea Carbonica; Causticum; Chamomilla; China; Carcinosin; Coffea; Lachesis; Lycopodium; Nux Vomica; Rhus Tox; Phosphorus; Pulsatilla; Thuja; Sulphur; Silica; Ignacia; Natrum Muriaticum.

Fevers (including infections, inflammation, viral, bacterial, malarial and nervous): Aconite; Arsenicum Album; Baptisia; Belladonna; China; Bryonia; Gelsemium; Hepar Sulphuricum; Lycopodium; Natrum Muriaticum; Nux Vomica; Phosphorus; Pyrogenium; Rhus Tox; Silica; Stramonium; Sulphur.

Organs (including liver, spleen, heart, kidney, bladder, brain and gallbladder): Arsenicum Album; Apis; Cantharis; Calcarea Carbonica; China; Ceanothus; Cardus Marianus; Alumina; Crataegus; Aurum; Berberis; Equisetum; Cheledonium; Lycopodium; Lachesis; Natrum Mur; Phosphorus; Nux Vomica; Belladonna.

The Mind (including anxiety, fears, confidence, anger, despair, confusion, blame, mental exhaustion, grief, guilt, mental restlessness, apathy, impatience, sensitive, stubborn, shy, suicidal and worried): Aconite; Aurum; Arsenicum Album; Argentum Nitricum; Causticum; Calcarea Carbonica; Calcarea Phosphoricum; Carcinosin; Kali Carbonicum; Ignacia; Lycopodium; Nux Vomica; Natrum Muriaticum; Natrum Phosphoricum; Mercurius; Nitricum Acidum; Phosphoric Acidum; Phosphorus; Stramonium; Silica; Sulphur; Thuja.

As mentioned earlier, there are over 2,800 proven remedies, and it would be impossible to include all of the appropriate ones in the headings just described. But, generally speaking, you will find that one or more of the remedies mentioned above are frequently included in a combination.

The main reason to take a formula or combination remedy is to get well or recover from an illness or accident. This recovery should be quick, painless and without side effects. Just as important for some is the low cost of the remedies in comparison to typical medical expenditures.

Using formula remedies essentially covers each

of these components, especially in acute or short-acting ailments. The remedy best suited to the illness is often found within the combination, as there may be up to 10 remedies combined in a formula. In effect, it is just the one that fits the disharmony that helps to alleviate it, while the others are rendered inert by the very effectiveness of the productive one.

An example of someone with allergies can demonstrate how this works. A 24-year-old woman has allergies to ragweed with the following symptoms: sneezing; burning, tearing eyes; itching throat; runny nose with a clear, watery discharge; head feels stuffy or congested; occasional wheezing with cough.

Combination remedies for allergies would generally include: Allium Cepa; Arsenicum Album; Euphrasia; Arundo; Wyethia; Sabadilla; Ambrosia; and possibly Nux Vomica, Arsenicum Iodatum or Natrum Muriaticum. There is one remedy that stands out above all the others and fits each of the allergic symptoms described in the example above, Ambrosia.

As Ambrosia so closely matches these symptoms, it eliminates them, brings about balance in the body and more or less negates the other listed remedies. Allergies disappear, the immune system becomes stronger and after a few more doses, the symptoms may not even return. All because the best suited remedy fit the symptom picture.

However, homeopathic remedies work because they relate to the symptoms, and the person, not because they are "magic pills." The body often takes a long time to recover balance, depending, of course, on the duration of illness. Remedies assist in accelerating the healing and balancing process, but not overnight. They work for the simple reason that they elevate the body to exert its fullest potential in recovery. But potential is rarely reached in a single day. Time and perseverance are part of the underlying principles of homeopathy, especially considering the time it takes to reach imbalance.

Combination remedies have a clear advantage over antacids, aspirin or other pain relievers, as they do not have side effects and can be just as potent. If the intent is to just get better for the moment, without considering the long term, then formula remedies are useful and relatively inexpensive. On the other hand, should your interest in healing be more permanent in nature, then the desired effects must consider deeper, single remedies.

Most of us take pills, whether they are medications, herbs or homeopathic remedies, to recover our health and eliminate the return of symptoms. Ragweed is more a trigger for allergic reactions than it is the actual cause. The specific cause can relate more to an oversensitive adrenal system, overuse of chemicals, inherited tendencies, processed foods, vaccinations or even pollution from the environment.

When we just treat allergic reactions, we do not alter the cause or replenish the adrenal system. We have a temporary resolution, and for some that is all that is needed. For others, elimination on a permanent basis is the ultimate desire. We are a nation desirous of the "quick fix," without consideration for the ill effects that such a "fix" has on the body.

Remember, use combinations for the short term and a single remedy for the long term or chronic illness. For help with the choice of single remedies, consult with a homeopath. Fortunately, homeopathic education has increased over the past decade and there are some excellent practitioners available in North America. Many are non-doctors who specialize in this growing field, which allows the costs to remain reasonable.

In 1990, there were over 37 million people who used alternative medical practices, and combination remedies were considered some of the safest and most reliable ones available. Traditional medicine does not effectively treat certain illnesses, or if it does, side effects are frequently greater than the disease.

A good example is the overuse of antibiotics for children with ear infections. After the antibiotic, the body's natural ability to combat bacteria is diminished and infections keep coming back. Combination remedies eliminate this type of recurrence and assist the body in preventing susceptibility to future disharmonies.

HOW TO USE HOMEOPATHIC REMEDIES

Homeopathic remedies in pill form look and taste like little sugar pills. They also come suspended in alcohol or other type of liquid dilution. When you take the pills, it is best not to touch them with your hands. Most homeopathic remedy containers provide a bottle cap or other type of top to make it easy for you to avoid touch-

ing the pills. Just pour the pills out into the top
and then directly into your mouth. The pills
should be dissolved in the mouth rather than
chewed or swallowed.

The liquid remedies can be dropped right on
the tongue (don't touch the dropper to your
mouth) or added to clean water.

The container will suggest the dose. Dosage is
not as important in homeopathy as getting the
right remedy. When you are self-treating, it is
probably best to use potencies of 6-30x or 6-
30c.

Most homeopaths recommend that you not eat
or drink anything within 20 or 30 minutes of taking a homeopathic remedy. While you are taking
a homeopathic remedy, you should not drink coffee or consume anything containing a strong essential oil such as eucalyptus, tea tree oil or
peppermint, menthol and camphor. Other things
that can "antidote" or cancel out the effectiveness of homeopathic remedies are drugs, nail
polish, and any type of strong negative emotional stress. People respond very differently to
homeopathic medicines: some are very sensitive
to them and may have them canceled out by
relatively minor tastes, smells or events, and in
others the remedies keep on working almost
regardless of what they do. I recommend you
keep a diary of what you notice and how
you're feeling.

Homeopathic combinations, when used as directed, and with proven remedies, are safe, effective and rarely have any side effects. You can feel
confident that this approach, which has been

used for over 200 years, effectively stimulates the immune system rather than diminishes it.

Homeopathy, whether used in combination or as a single remedy, assists the body in rediscovering its natural ability to heal itself. Few other approaches to healing can make that same claim.

CHAPTER 3

62 of the Most Commonly Prescribed Homeopathic Remedies

This chapter is a listing of 62 homeopathic remedies and their "symptoms," as described by homeopath David Dancu. They are only a small portion of the 2,800 remedies available, but they will give you a very good sense of what is available, and what types of symptoms to look for in a homeopathic treatment. According to Dancu, some 70 to 80 percent of all disharmonies treated with homeopathy will be well-served by using one of these remedies. Use this as a general guide, and as a way to familiarize yourself with the essence and identity of each remedy.

Studying and understanding homeopathic remedies is a long-term process. Many remedies have similar traits and symptoms, but each has some unique component to set it apart from the others. These are the aspects that give a deeper comprehension of its essence and help establish a better grasp of the whole remedy.

Aconite: worse after cold, wet weather; anxiety and fears; shock; panic attacks; early or sudden onset of illness; restlessness.

Alumina: anxiety from being hurried; dullness; mental slowness; dryness of all membranes; constipation; disorientation; dizziness; itchiness of the skin without eruptions.

Anacardium: low self-esteem; abusive; cursing; depression; fears and delusions; controlling; violent and angry; brain fatigue; most symptoms are better from eating; strong sexual desires.

Apis: redness, itching, swelling; busy; thirstless; right-sided ailments; worse from heat applications.

Argentum Nitricum: anxiety and panic attacks; impulsive; feelings of abandonment; open and excitable; warm blooded; worse eating sweets, but craves them; gastrointestinal problems; left sided ailments; many phobias.

Arnica: trauma and injuries; concussions; bruises; irritability; prefers to be alone; relief of pains; refuses doctor's help.

Arsenicum Album: anxiety; restlessness; avarice; compulsive; fearful; depressed; skin disharmonies; chilly; controlling without spontaneity; right-sided ailments; worse around midnight; asthma; thirst for small sips; burning sensations.

Aurum: severe suicidal depression; serious; self-condemnation; guilt and abandonment issues; worse cloudy weather; intense; worse with pain; anger with remorse; moans during sleep.

Baryta Carbonica: slowness in mental development; immature behavior; low self-esteem; shy and yielding; anxious and nervous; chronic tonsillitis; blank facial expression.

Belladonna: early onset with redness, heat, flushing of the face and fever; delirium; anger intense with hitting, biting; migraines; thirstless; strep and sore throats.

Bryonia: worse with any movement/motion; irritability; prefers solitude; fear of business or financial failure; dry mucus membranes and dry colon; intense thirst; warm blooded; joint problems.

Calcarea Carbonica: overly responsible; bone problems; fear of heights; fear of going insane; overwhelmed; slow development as a child; stubborn; overweight; slow metabolism; head sweats; milk allergy.

Calcarea Phosphorica: complains about everything; loves change and travel; dissatisfied; sensitive; craves smoked foods; state of weakness; grief with sighing; slow development.

Cantharis: urinary tract infections; burning sensations; strong sexual desires; incontinence; violent emotions.

Carbo Vegetabilise: intense irritability; gastrointestinal problems; negative; prostration and weakness; coma; indifference; coldness; air hunger.

Carcinosin: intense, sympathetic, passionate; family history of cancer; fastidious; craves chocolate and spicy food; moles on back; strong libido; loves animals; low energy from 3 to 6 p.m.; loves travel.

Causticum: idealistic and rebellious; sympathetic; serious; very sensitive to suffering of others; grief;

joint and TMJ problems; warts; compulsive; desires smoked foods; chilly; incontinence.

Chamomilla: peevish when ill; intense irritability; excessive sensitivity to pains; infant desires to be carried; one cheek red, other pale; colic; ear infections; teething problems; worse with travel.

China Officinalis: internal sensitivity; introverted; taciturn; gastrointestinal disharmonies; worse loss of fluids; anemia; colitis; worse touch; periodicity of complaints; fear of animals.

Conium: emotional flatness or indifference; paralysis; cancer; hardness of glands; tumors; fixed ideas; fogginess of the brain.

Cuprum: spasms and convulsions; appears emotionally closed; sensation of suffocating; flat facial expression; seizures; rigid; intense emotions suppressed.

Ferrum Metallicum: anemia; desires raw meat; overweight; face flushes easily; very sensitive to noise; strong willed; better walking slowly; general weakness and fatigue; demanding.

Gelsemium: fatigue; heaviness of the eyelids; brain fatigue; stage fright; weakness of will; cowardly; indifference; forgetful; tremble with anticipation; depressed; thirstless; chilly; headaches; diarrhea.

Graphites: slowness with poor concentration; skin abnormalities; irritable; anxious; herpes; indecisive; many self-doubts; fastidious; overweight tendencies; offensive sweats; restlessness; photophobia.

Hepar Sulphuris: anger when security is threatened; irritable; worse any draft of air; sensitive; chilly; infections and abscesses; intense and hurried; rarely cheerful; abusive; overreacts to pains.

Hyoscyamus: paranoia; jealous with violent outbursts; intense sexual desires; worse with touch; hyperactive child; shameless; defiant; delusions; talkative; fear of dogs; wild gestures.

Ignacia: acute grief or worse since grief; romantic/idealistic; aggravation from consolation; prefers to be alone; stress is better after eating; better with exercise; sighing; disappointed love.

Iodum: very warm; thyroid dysfunctions; very restless and busy; compulsive; talkative and anxious; impulsive; intense appetite; anger; avoids company; discontent and destruction; general fears.

Kali Bichromicum: sinus disharmonies/headaches; strong sense of right and wrong; thick, yellow, ropy discharges; rigid and proper; self-occupied; suppresses emotional aspects of personality.

Kali Carbonicum: righteousness and strong sense of duty; mind rules emotions; fear of losing control; rigid; asthma; possessive; conservative; quarrelsome; self-reproach; worse 2 to 5 a.m.

Lachesis: left-sided complaints; loquacity; suspicious; jealous; sarcastic; opinionated and can be fanatical; warm blooded; all types of menstrual disharmonies; intense personality; vindictive; active mind; drug and alcohol addictions; low self-esteem.

Ledum: prefers solitude; hatred for self and others; joint problems; worse heat, although chilly;

worse movement or motion; irritable; insect bites, lockjaw, or injuries with bruising; puncture wounds.

Lycopodium: poor self-confidence; anger and irritability; liver and kidney disharmonies; fears and anxieties; hyperactive children; right-sided ailments; low energy 4 to 8 p.m.; anticipatory anxiety; tendency to dominate or control; opinionated; avoids responsibility; digestive problems; generally chilly but prefers open air and worse warmth.

Magnesia Muriatica: yielding; aversion to confrontations; feels anxious at night; very responsible; noises annoy; composed, with suppressed inner anger; depression; unrefreshing sleep.

Medorrhinum: nasal discharges; cruel and aggressive behavior; an extremist; "sex, drugs, and rock 'n' roll;" self-centered and loves danger; obsessive/compulsive; history of VD; hurried; intense passions; bites fingernails; overwhelmed by impulses; night person; loves sea.

Mercurius: strong reaction to temperature changes; emotionally closed; stammering speech; conservative; anxious with destructive ideas; paranoia; facade; worse at night; excess saliva; night sweats; serious appearance; metallic taste in mouth; gum infections.

Natrum Carbonicum: very sensitive; craves potatoes; inner turmoil and depression with appearance of cheerfulness; prefers solitude; emotionally closed; sweet and selfless; delicate; poor digestion; worse heat and sun; sadness; milk allergies; sympathetic.

Natrum Muriaticum: fear of being hurt; closed emotionally from past grief; very sensitive; critical; perfectionist; romantic; strong desire for solitude; serious and controlled; introverted; depression; generally worse from being in the sun or heat; hay fever; herpes.

Natrum Sulphuricum: head injuries and concussions; suicidal depressions; very responsible and serious; warm blooded; feels better after a bowel movement; emotionally closed; asthma; possible past history of venereal disease; sensitive; practical, with business focus.

Nitricum Acidum: generally negative person; self-discontent and anger; curses; restless; hypersensitive; selfish; anxieties about health and death; vindictive; chilly pains come and go suddenly.

Nux Vomica: Type "A" personality; ambitious; meticulous; hypersensitive, with tendency to over-react; liver and bowel remedy; driven to excess; addictive personality; sensitive nervous system; intense irritation from wind; chilly; increased hunger.

Petroleum: skin disharmonies of all types, with dryness; quick temper; motion sickness; herpes; offensive perspiration; unable to make decisions; chilly; worse in winter; increased hunger.

Phosphoricum Acidum: dullness and slowness; apathy; feels overwhelmed with grief and emotions; intense fatigue and loss of energy; yielding; desires refreshing fruits; dehydration; chilly.

Phosphorus: expressive and extroverted; prefers consolation and company; impressionable and very sensitive; many fears and anxieties; affectionate; chilly, yet likes cold drinks; craves spicy, salty and sweets; sympathetic; intuitive; nosebleeds.

Platinum: primarily a female remedy; haughty to the extreme; is worse with touch; idealistic; dwells on the past; feels abandoned; dislikes children; insolent and rude; pretentious; strong libido.

Plumbum: taciturn; sad; shy; selfish; difficulty in expressing themselves; indifference; illness slow in development; very chilly; pains tend to radiate; neurological disorders.

Psorinum: skin dysfunction of all types; periodicity; pessimist; tend to despair with hopelessness; anxiety and fear, especially of poverty; very chilly; low energy; feels forsaken/lost; dirty skin.

Pulsatilla: warm-blooded; capricious mood swings; PMS; mild and dependent nature; female remedy; abandonment issues; desires consolation; weepy; digestive and sinus (thick yellow/green mucus) problems; worse heat and craves fresh air; thirstless with dryness.

Rhus Toxicodendron: great internal restlessness; obsessive tendencies; skin and joint remedy; feels better stretching and with motion; withhold affections/feelings; apprehensive at night; timid; herpes with burning and itching; worse cold/damp.

Ruta: affects tendons and fibrous tissues; distrustful; startles easily; argumentative; stiffness/pain; strains; sprains; eyestrain; related headaches; worse motion or lying on painful side.

Sepia: indifference and desire to be alone; impatience; irritability; low sexual desires; chilly; grief and depression; PMS/menopause; bearing down sensations; leucorrhea; taciturn and negative; herpes.

Silica: yielding; timid and bashful; emotionally dependent; low self-esteem; stubborn; chilly; conscientious about details; constipation; slow development; weakness; perspires easily; recurring infections.

Spigelia: left sided ailments; serious; responsible; violent pains; migraines; grief; worse tobacco smoke; anxiety of pointed objects; pinworms; combination heart and eye symptoms; chilly; worse touch.

Spongia: fear of suffocation; heart ailments; increased anxiety; dry mucus membranes; dry, barking, croupy cough; easily frightened; thyroid disharmonies; respiratory conditions; weakness.

Staphysagria: sweet, yielding person; suppressed emotions; very sensitive; emotionally dependent; fear of losing control; possible history of sexual abuse or humiliation; strong sexual history; grief; suppressed anger; low self-confidence; worse after nap; mild.

Stramonium: violent tendencies; etiology from a fright; impulsive rage; wild behavior; night terror; desires company and light; intense thirst; flushed face; excitable; stammers; convulsions; promiscuous; hyperactive children; could be mild, gentle and very sensitive.

Sulphur: idealistic and philosophical; self-contained; indolent; warm blooded; burning sensations; desires spicy foods; appearance is not important; collect things; opinionated; desires open air; itch; offensive discharges; offended by others' body odor; aversion to bathing.

Syphilinum: compulsive tendencies; worse at night; very chilly; alcoholic; excess saliva; fear of disease/germs or going insane; nails are distorted; anxious; indifferent; worse hot or cold extremes.

Thuja: low self-confidence; emotionally closed and hard to get to know; secretive; fastidious; hurried; herpes and suppressed venereal disease; ailments after vaccinations; urine stream is forked; runny nose with stool; chilly; left sided ailments; irritable; warts; oily skin.

Tuberculinum: desires change and travel; feels unfulfilled; can be mean; compulsive; chilly; respiratory disharmonies; milk and cat allergies; hyperactive children; romantic longings; desires smoked foods; excess perspiration at night; itch, better with heat.

Veratrum Album: self-righteous and haughty; thinking more than feeling; precocious child; hyperactive child; ambitious; deceitful; very chilly; abusive spouse; critical; jealous; restlessness; religious mania; excessive cold sweats; inappropriate kissing or hugging.

Zincum: hypersensitive and overstimulated; impulsive movements; restlessness; always complaining; mentally overwhelmed and fatigued; worse when drinking wine or alcohol; superstitious; chilly; affected by noises; feels better after eating.

CHAPTER 4

Remedies for Short-Term, Acute Illnesses

Homeopathic self-treatment and combination remedies are best suited to acute illnesses. An acute illness is self-limiting, meaning that it has a life span of approximately seven to ten days. Without any treatment, it usually goes away on its own. The following chapter is a compilation of the most common acute remedies as compiled by homeopath, teacher and author David Dancu.

Homeopathy is not used for every symptom that arises, as these symptoms are the body's messages of disharmony. A fever is a message that there is an infection and body heat is a means of disarming or eliminating the infection. By allowing the body to function as much as possible without outside influences, it finds a way to recover and regain its energy, balance and strength.

The following list of remedies covers a variety of acute illnesses along with some proven remedies. These brief symptoms will help you in using homeopathy for short-term acute illnesses and can be helpful in some emergencies. Obviously, if there is a crisis or critical situation, common sense dictates that proper medical treatment be obtained. On the other hand, homeopathic remedies are excellent for shock and emergencies while a person is being transported to the hospital or health care provider.

ACCIDENTS

Abrasions/cuts

Arnica for trauma of all types and bleeding, even coma.
Calendula for antiseptic use, either internal or external.
Hypericum for injury to nerve endings or incisions.
Ledum helps heal puncture and penetration wounds.

Burns

Cantharis reduces pain and promotes healing process.
Urtica Urens for first- and second-degree burns.
Hypericum reduces pain when nerve endings are involved such as spine, fingers and teeth.
Belladonna for fever, flushing of the face and delirium.

Bites

Ledum for all types of bites with coldness around area.
Hypericum when pain seems excessive for the wound.
Belladonna for dog and snake bites.
Lachesis for snake bites or with flushes of heat.

Bruises

Arnica for bruises or muscle injuries.
Bellis for trauma, contusions and soreness.
Hamamelis helps with internal bleeding and bruising.
Ruta for stiffness in muscles and tendons from bruising.

Bleeding

Phosphorus for all types of hemorrhaging.
Ferrum Phosphoricum helps coagulate the blood.
Lachesis when blood is dark and area is blue.
Ipecacuanha for gushing, bright red blood with nausea.

Head Injuries

Arnica for all types; conscious or unconscious.
Cicuta for dilated pupils, muscle spasms and stiffness.
Gelsemium for occipital pain and heaviness of the eyes.
Hypericum for numbness, tingling and seizures.

Shock

Aconite after sudden fright or fearful situation.
Arnica after an injury or trauma, causing shock.
Carbo Vegetabilis for fainting, coldness and difficulty breathing.
Veratrum Album when skin and perspiration are very cold.

Whiplash

Bryonia when any movement is painful.
Causticum when neck muscles and tendons contract.
Hypericum if nerves and a tingling sensation are involved.
Rhus Tox for injuries that are better with motion and heat.

ALLERGIES

Anaphylactic Shock

Apis for constriction, inflammation, swelling, hives, redness of the skin and soreness; worse with heat.
Urtica Urens for eruptions, itching, blotches and burning; heat with a stinging sensation.
Consider: Arsenicum Album; Natrum Mur; Rhus Tox.

To Animals

Arsenicum Album for respiratory-related reactions.
Allium Cepa for clear, burning nasal discharge with runny eyes.
Euphrasia for profuse, burning discharge from eyes.
Natrum Mur for egg white-like discharge; cannot smell.
Consider: Sabadilla, Nux Vomica; Tuberculinum; Sulphur.

To Chemicals

Arsenicum when there is a burning sensation after exposure.

Coffea for excitability of the mind and nervousness.

Mercurius when you feel worse at night with excess sweat.

Nitricum Acid for the oversensitive, depressed and negative types.

Consider: Nux Vomica, Phosphorus; Sulphur; Psorinum.

To Dust

Arsenicum Album when respiration/wheezing is involved.

Bromium when there is a feeling of suffocation and coldness.

Hepar for heart palpitations and anxious wheezing.

Consider: Silica; Ipecacuanha; Pothos.

To Foods

Beans: Bryonia; Lycocpodium; Petroleum; Calcarea Carb.

Bread: Bryonia; Lycopodium; Natrum Mur; Pulsatilla; Sepia.

Cheese: Arsenicum; Nux Vomica; Phosphorus; Sepia.

Coffee: Cantharis; Causticum; Chamomilla; Nux Vomica.

Fruit: Arsenicum; Bryonia; China; Colocynthis; Pulsatilla.

Meat: Arsenicum; Calcarea; China; Ferrum; Kali Carb.

Milk: Calcarea; China; Magnesium Mur; Natrum Carb; Sepia.
Onions: Lycopodium; Thuja; Sulphur; Ignacia; Pulsatilla.
Potatoes: Aluminum; Bryonia; Silica; Sepia; Pulsatilla.
Salt: Carbo Vegetabilis; Natrum Mur; Drosera; Phosphorus; Silica.
Starches: Berberis; Lycopodium; Natrum Mur; Lachesis.
Sugar: Argentum Nit; Lycopodium; Sulphur; Phosphorus.
Vegetables: Aluminum; Bryonia; Kali Carb; Natrum Sulph.
Wheat: Allium cepa; Lycopodium; Natrum Mur; Pulsatilla.

Hay Fever

Arsenicum Iod. for profuse watery discharges and tickling.
Wyethia for itching of the palate and dry mucous membranes.
Arundo for burning and itch in nostrils with sneezing.
Arum for sneezing and tickling sensations; congestion.
Consider: Arsenicum; Allium Cepa; Sabadilla; Euphrasia.

Insect Bites

Ledum for any puncture wound with coldness around the wound.
Apis for red, hot, swollen skin that is worse with heat.

Hypericum for tingling sensations or numbness.
Urtica Urens for hives, itching, redness and worse with heat.
Consider: Arsenicum; Belladonna; Thuja; Lachesis.

Poison Ivy

Bryonia has swelling, heat, dryness, thirst and is irritable.
Anacardium for intense itch with swelling and redness.
Croton Tig. for painful scratching and pustules; intense.
Graphites for a watery discharge from the reaction.
Consider: Clematis; Rhus Tox; Sepia; Sanguianaria.

To Smoke

Euphrasia for burning in the eyes and nasal discharge.
Ignacia when breathing is affected; person feels annoyed.
Sepia for nausea and exhaustion with any left-sidedness.
Spigelia for dryness, tickling and constriction in throat.
Consider: Nux Vomica; Natrum Mur; Causticum; Sulphur.

CHILDREN'S REMEDIES

Colic

Chamomilla desires to be carried, is irritable and angry.

Colocynthis for a bloated stomach with intense pains.
Dioscorea for arching back with cramping pains and gas.
Magnesia Phos when a child feels better bending double with the cramps.

Chicken Pox

Aconite for the first stages of the outbreak.
Antimonium Crudum when overheated and angry.
Rhus Tox for restless, intense itch with swollen glands.
Sulphur for a burning itch which is worse in heat and sweat.

Colds

Aconite for sudden onset from cold, dry winds.
Belladonna for early stage with fever, redness and thirst.
Kali Bic when discharge is thick yellow/green and ropy.
Pulsatilla for thick yellow mucus and clinging to parent.
Consider: Allium Cepa; Euphrasia; Hepar; Nux Vomica.

Coughs

Barking: Aconite; Belladonna; Drosera; Spongia.
Croupy: Aconite; Hepar Sulphuris; Spongia; Lachesis; Phos.
Dry: Belladonna; Bryonia; Drosera; Natrum Mur; Rumex.

Hacking: Allium Cepa; Arsenicum; Drosera; Phosphorus.
Rattling: Antimonium Tart; Causticum; Dulcamura; Ipecacuanha.
Violent: Belladonna; Causticum; Cuprum; Lachesis; Phosphorus.
Whooping: Antimonium Tart; Carbo Vegetabilis; Cuprum; Drosera.

Diarrhea

Arsenicum for a watery, burning stool with nausea.
China for a painless stool containing undigested food.
Podophyllum for a frequent, gushing stool that is smelly.
Rheum for sour smelling stool resulting from teething.
Consider: Nux Vomica, Sulphur; Silica; Rhus Tox.

Earache

Aconite for the early stages with cold symptoms.
Chamomilla when pain and irritability arise together.
Hepar for smelly discharges; is worse when cold.
Pulsatilla for congestion with redness and discharge.
Consider: Lycopodium; Silica; Mercurius; Belladonna.

Fevers

Aconite for sudden onset with anxiety, heat and dryness.

Belladonna for flushed face, burning heat and delirium.

Gelsemium for shivering, heat, drowsiness and no sweat.

Mercurius for excess saliva; heat alternates with chills.

Consider: Natrum Mur; Nux Vomica; Pulsatilla; Sulphur.

Influenza

Oscillococcinum for the earliest stages, within 24 hours.

Baptisia for prostration, muscle soreness and stomach.

Eupatorium when there is deep bone ache and debility.

Gelsemium for drowsiness, aches, chills and exhaustion.

Consider: Arsenicum; Bryonia; Rhus Tox; Nux Vomica.

Indigestion

China when gas arises after eating fruit; bloated.

Ignacia when problem is caused by any type of emotional upset.

Lycopodium for gas and bloating made worse by eating.

Nux Vomica from overindulgence of food or drink.

Consider: Argentum Nitninme; Pulsatilla; Carbo Vegetabilis; Sulphur.

Measles

Aconite is excellent for early stages.
Belladonna for fever; is used in the early stages.
Bryonia for cough, fever, dryness and intense thirst.
Pulsatilla is restless and desires attention; no thirst.
Consider: Gelsemium; Apis; Euphrasia; Phosphorus.

Mumps

Belladonna for swelling, fever, heat and redness.
Jaborandi for redness, swollen glands and excess saliva.
Mercurius for painful swelling, fever and profuse sweat.
Rhus Tox for swelling with fever; better with heat.
Consider: Aconite, Apis; Lachesis; Phytolacca; Pulsatilla.

Rash (Diaper)

Apis for red, sore, shiny and hot skin; worse with heat.
Petroleum for dry, red, itching and cracked skin.
Rhus Tox when it is better with hot baths; skin itches, flakes and burns.
Sulphuricum Acidum for blotchy, red skin; worse with heat.
Consider: Sulphur; Graphites; Mezereum; Urtica Urens.

Sore Throat

Aconite for heat and fever from dry cold winds.
Belladonna is the first choice with heat and redness.
Causticum for burning, soreness, rawness and tightness.
Phytolacca for congestion, redness and very painful.
Consider: Apis; Hepar; Lachesis; Mercurius; Gelsemium.

Teething

Belladonna for pain, fever, shrieking, restless and flushed.
Calcarea Phos for slow, difficult dentition.
Chamomilla for intense pain, irritability and hot cheeks.
Pulsatilla for clinginess; painful dentition. Better in fresh air.
Consider: Coffea; Silica; Kreosotum; Rheum; Phytolacca.

HEADACHES

Migraine:

Bryonia for a pressing sensation with thirst; worse with motion.
Gelsemium for dull, droopy mind fog; blurred vision.
Glonoinium for throbbing pain, heaviness and irritability.

Melilotus for bursting pain with red face and nausea.

Sanguinaria for right-sided pain that radiates to eye; worse in the a.m.

Consider: Belladonna; Iris; Coffea; Apis; Nux Vomica; Spigelia.

Tension

Argentum Nitricum for an enlarged head feeling with impulsiveness.

Ignacia when you feel worse from any emotional stress or anxiety.

Natrum Mur feels like pounding hammers; worse 10:00 a.m.; throbs.

Phosphoric Acid when apathetic; worse from loss of fluids or emotions.

Zincum when exhausted, nervous and restless; noise sensitive.

Consider: Coffea; Gelsemium; China; Nux Vomica; Thuja; Phos.

Hormonal

Cyclamen for a flickering sensation; worse in open air and when chilled.

Kreosotum for menstrual headaches with irritability.

Lachesis for deep pain, coming in waves; left-sided with burning.

Sepia feels as if there is a band around the head; left side; sad.

Pulsatilla for when you feel weepy, sad, thirstless and are sweating; better in open air.

Consider: Lycopodium; Natrum Mur; Belladonna; Lac Caninum.

Sick

Cocculus for motion sickness, loss of sleep or noise.

Chelidonium for liver-related and right-sided sickness with drowsiness.

Nux Vomica for overindulgence of any kind.

Picric Acid for mental strain, fatigue or travel.

Consider: Iris; Ipecacuanha; Sulphur; Arsenicum Album; Sanguinaria.

Sinus

Dulcamara for changes in barometric pressure; worse in damp air.

Euphrasia for burning sensation in the eyes with tearing.

Kali Bic for burning sensation at root of nose; pain in one area; sinusitis.

Mercurius for excess saliva, bad breath and metallic taste.

Consider: Calcarea Sulph; Hepar; Nux Vomica; Thuja; Natrum Mur.

Periodic

Arsenicum for one specific time of day with burning; better with heat.

China when worse from loss of fluids or malaria; liver ailments.

Nitricum Acidum for burning nasal discharge; worse with pressure.

Silica for radiating pains, head sweats, worse drafts, chills.

Consider: Natrum Mur; Sanguinaria; Sepia; Lachesis; Ignacia.

SPORTS INJURIES

Broken Bones/Fractures

Arnica for the earliest stage of trauma or injury.
Bryonia when pain is intense from any type of motion.
Calcarea Phos helps in formation of callus in fractures.
Symphytum helps bones to properly knit after being set.
Consider: Hypericum; Rhus Tox; Ruta; Silica; Calcarea.

Dislocations

Carbo Animalis for diminished strength and tendon contraction.
Kali Nitricum for numbness, heaviness and weakness of limbs.
Calcarea when the problem is chronic and fails to heal.
Ruta when tendons are involved, especially wrist and ankle.
Consider: Arnica; Natrum Carb; Rhus Tox; Lycopodium; Bryonia.

Pulled Hamstring

Bellis for soreness, stiffness, coldness and bruising.

Ambra-G for drawing pain; limb seems shortened; tingling.

Causticum for hardness of tendons and contractions; cramps.

Ledum for swelling and stiffness; better with ice.

Consider: Arnica; Ruta; Rhus Tox; Bryonia; Sulphuricum Acidum.

Hip Pointers

Aesculus for radiating pain that is worse upon standing.

Calcarea Phos for stiffness; worse with motion or air drafts.

Rhus Tox if stretching reduces pain; better with heat.

Ruta for lameness and stiffness; better when lying down.

Consider: Arnica; Bellis; Hamamelis; Symphytum; Bryonia.

Sprains/Strains

Bryonia when worse from any movement; wants to be alone.

Bellis for stiffness with a bruised sensation.

Asafoetida for hysteria with bone pains and inflammation.

Millefolium for tearing pains from overexertion; irritable.

Consider: Arnica (first); Rhus Tox; Ruta; Ledum.

TRAVEL

Constipation

Alumina when patient has no desire for stool or may strain; straining; worse with travel.

Bryonia for dark, dry, hard stool; very thirsty for cold water.

Nux Vomica when bloated and irritable; never feels fully vacated.

Silica for ineffectual urging; hard stool which pulls back in.

Consider: Plumbum; Sulphur; Opium; Aloe; Sepia; Nitricum Acidum.

Diarrhea

Aconite after cold, dry wind or fright.

Arsenicum for prostration, vomiting, restlessness and anxiety.

China after eating fruit or a summer chill; painless; fever.

Colocynthis for intense colicky pains; better with pressure.

Consider: Nux Vomica; Veratrum Album; Podophyllum; Aloe; Sulphur.

Indigestion

Anacardium for heartburn two hours after eating; pain/fullness.

Carbo Vegetabilis for offensive gas, bloating, pain and internal heat.

Lycopodium when bloated with pain; better after passing gas.

Nux Vomica when worse after overeating; gas, bloating and cramping.

Consider: Arsenicum; Bryonia; China; Pulsatilla; Sulphur; Hepar.

Influenza/Cold

Ferrum Phos for the earliest stages without clear symptoms.
Baptisia for prostration, cramps, nausea and confusion.
Gelsemium when achy, chilled, weak and anxious; heavy eyelids.
Eupatorium Perf. for deep bone aches with chills and headache.
Consider: Arsenicum; Bryonia; Nux Vomica; Rhus Tox; Hepar.

Jet Lag

Cocculus when lack of sleep causes irritability and fatigue.
Gelsemium for heavy eyes, headache, weakness and tired limbs.
Argentum Nitricum for fear and panic while flying; anxious.
Arnica for being cramped in a seat for a long period.
Consider: Rescue Remedy; Phos Acid; Zincum; Sulphuricum Acidum.

Motion Sickness

Borax for nausea or vomiting; worse with downward motion.
Cocculus for queasiness; worse with the thought of food.
Nux Vomica for nausea, headache and chills; no desire for food.

Tabacum when chilled, giddy and sweating; worse with tobacco smoke.
Consider: Rhus Tox; Petroleum; Ipecacuanha.

Sleeplessness

Arsenicum for restlessness, anxiety, fatigue and irritability.
Coffea when nervous, anxious, hypersensitive and mentally active.
Ignacia when worse from emotional stress or grief.
Nux Vomica when worse from overeating, alcohol or mental strain.
Consider: Aconite; Lycopodium; Pulsatilla; Arnica.

Stress

Natrum Mur for long-term emotional ill effects and solitude.
Nux Vomica when there is mental stress and overstimulation.
Passiflora when overworked, worried, restless and exhausted.
Valerian when oversensitive, irritable, nervous and changeable.
Consider: Zincum; Arsenicum; Argent Nit; Ignacia; Sepia.

WOMEN'S AILMENTS

Cystitis

Apis for burning, stinging and soreness when urinating.
Cantharis for intense urging, burning which is passed by drops.

Equisetum for bladder fullness, severe pain and frequent urge.

Lycopodium for low back pains, straining and retention.

Consider: Aconite; Belladonna; Lachesis; Sepia; Pulsatilla.

Discharges

Black: China; Kreosotum; Rhus Tox; Secale.

Bloody: Calcarea Sulph; China; Cocculus; Nitricum Acidum; Sepia.

Burning: Calcarea; Borax; Kreosotum; Pulsatilla; Sulphur.

Green: Carbo Vegetabilis; Kali Bic; Mercurius; Natrum Mur; Sepia.

Itching: Calcarea; China; Mercurius; Sepia; Kreosotum; Zincum.

Milky: Calcarea; Kali Mur; Sepia; Silica; Pulsatilla; Lachesis.

Offensive: Kali Arsenicum; Kreosotum; Mercurius; Nux Vomica.

Profuse: Calcarea; Graphites; Sepia; Silica; Stannum; Thuja.

Thick: Arsenicum; Calcarea; Kali Bic; Natrum Carb; Thuja; Zinc

Thin: Graphites; Nitricum Acidum; Pulsatilla; Sulphur; Silica; Sepia.

White: Borax; Graphites; Natrum Mur; Sepia; Nux Vomica; Pulsatilla.

Yellow: Arsenicum; Calcarea; Chamomilla; Hydrastis; Pulsatilla.

Genital Herpes

Natrum Mur for tingling sensations; worse in sun or under stress.

Petroleum for sensations of moisture with crusting and itch.

Sepia for itching, worse at folds of skin and in spring; odor.

Thuja for eruptions on covered parts only; sensitive to touch.

Consider: Rhus Tox; Alnus; Medorrhinum; Lachesis; Dulcamura.

Menopause

Lachesis for hot flashes and fainting; worse with tight clothing.

Lilium Tig for intensity, depression, irritability and prolapsed.

Pulsatilla when clingy, complaining, weepy and sad; worse with heat.

Sepia when overwhelmed and irritable; prefers solitude; hot flashes.

Consider: Sulphur; Natrum Mur; Phosphorus; Sabina; Kreosotum.

Menses

Absent: Aurum; Ferrum; Graphites; Kali Carb; Lycopodium; Pulsatilla.

Clotted: Belladonna; Calcarea; China; Lachesis; Sabina; Pulsatilla.

Cramps: Chamomilla; Cocculus; Colocynthis; Mag Phos; Sepia.

Frequent: Arsenicum; Belladonna; Cyclamen; Ferrum Phos.

Irregular: Argent Nit; Nux Moschata; Pulsatilla; Sepia; Senecio.

Late: Causticum; Cuprum; Lachesis; Natrum Mur; Sarsaparilla.

Painful: Cimicifuga; Mag Phos; Millefolium; Cactus; Pulsatilla; Sabina; Sulphur; Caulophyllum; Cyclamen; Chamomilla.
Profuse: Arsenicum; Ferrum Phos; Phos; Calcarea Phos; Sabina; Senecio; Millefolium; Natrum Mur; Ferrum; Cyclamen.
Suppressed: Belladonna; Cyclamen; Lachesis; Senecio; Sepia.

Pelvic Inflammatory Disease

Arsenicum for burning, offensive discharge with anxiety.
Lac Caninum for ovarian pains and vaginal gas; fear of snakes.
Lachesis for left-sided pains and cysts; worse with tight clothing.
Sabina for severe PMS, intense pains, gushing flow; leucorrhea.
Consider: Apis; Belladonna; Cantharis; Pulsatilla; Chamomilla; Sepia.

Vaginitis

Medorrhinum for high sex drive and chronic infection; herpes.
Pulsatilla when needy and capricious; does not tolerate pain.
Thuja for green discharges, herpes, polyps and cysts.
Kreosotum for strong itch with burning discharge and odor.
Consider: Arsenicum; Graphites; Mercurius; Sepia; Sulphur.

CHAPTER 5

The Homeopathic First Aid Kit

Many homeopathic remedies are useful as immediate treatment in the case of injury or accident. Homeopathic treatment for emergencies does not require the detailed taking of a case needed for chronic illnesses. Only a small number of remedies apply. It is important to remember that homeopathic medicines should not be used in place of standard first aid measures. Always perform these procedures first and summon help when needed.

For on-the-spot treatment, besides pellets and tablets, homeopathic tinctures can be applied directly to injured sites. Tinctures are prepared with alcohol which can sting cuts and broken skin.

It's always worth using topical applications made from the original substances of certain homeopathic remedies such as calendula. The creams and lotions make very effective support for remedies taken internally.

FIRST AID DOSES

Common dosage of homeopathic remedies in first aid is two tablets, three to four times a day. This can increase to two tablets every 30 minutes to one hour when pain is severe. Reduce the frequency as improvement begins, but continue dosing until improvement is well established.

Remedy	Used for	Benefits
Arnica (Internal and as oil or ointment. Use before other remedies to treat the shock of any injury.)	Bleeding under skin Bruises, ordinary Burns (Treatment for shock only) Fractures Injuries from blows or falls Bee, hornet and wasp stings Jagged cuts (internal remedy only) Muscular soreness Shin splints Shock Soreness, general Strains, general Strained back muscles Twisted knee (Take on first day)	Speeds healing. Relieves pain. Reduces swelling.
Bryonia	Injured joint (swollen, distended, worse with movement) Twisted knee (take on 2nd day if worse with movement) Fractured ribs	Relieves pain. Speeds healing.
Calendula (Nonalcoholic lotion for cuts or ointment for scrapes,	Abrasions Bee, hornet and wasp stings Bleeding from mouth Burns, 1st degree (add	Cleanses and speeds healing of slight wounds. Helps stop

etc. Saturate dressing with lotion. (Lotion or ointment)	drops to cold water treatment.) Jock itch Scratches Superficial wounds	bleeding. Inhibits infection.
Cantharis	Burns, 3rd degree (internally only)	Speeds healing.
Glonoinium	Sunstroke and heat exhaustion	Speeds recovery.
Hypericum (Lotion for external use)	Crushed nerves Burns, 2nd degree (Immerse in lotion) Nerve injuries to extremities and elbows Puncture wounds	Promotes tissue growth. Speeds healing. Relieves pain.
Ledum (Lotion for external use)	Bee, hornet, wasp stings Bruises (cold, numb, long-lasting) Black eye Puncture wounds Splinter under nail Swelling	Reduces pain and inflammation, especially when wound relieved by cold.
Rhus Toxicodendron (Use after Arnica)	Blistery itches Injury after lifting/ overexertion Joints, creaky Joints, hot, swollen Strained/torn muscles, tendons, ligaments Poison Ivy/Oak Tendonitis	Relieves aches and itching. Speeds healing.

Ruta   Bruised bone covering   Speeds
(Use after   Injuries to bones   healing.
Arnica and   Lame feeling
when Rhus   Prolapsed, protruding
Tox has not   rectum
helped)   Soft tissue injuries
                              Sprains to ankle/wrist
                              Strained/torn muscles
                              (when initial swelling
                              has decreased)

RESOURCES AND REFERENCES

David A. Dancu, N.D. is a practicing homeopath who teaches and has a private practice in Boulder, Colorado. His new book, *Homeopathic Vibrations . . . A Guide for Natural Healing* (Sunshine Press, 1996) is available through book stores or by mail for $22.95 (P.O. Box 333, Hygiene, CO 80533).

Bellavite, P., Signorini, A., *Homeopathy, A Frontier in Medical Science*, North Atlantic Books, Calif., 1995.

Boericke & Tafel, *The Family Guide to Self-medication, Homeopathic*, Boericke & Tafel, Inc., Calif. 1988.

Cummings, S., Ullman, D., *Everybody's Guide to Homeopathic Medicines*, G.P. Putnam's Sons, New York, 1991.

Dancu, D.A., *Homeopathic Vibrations, A Guide to Natural Healing*, Sunshine Press, Boulder, Colo., 1996.

Hamilton, S., "What You Should Know About Homeopathy," *American Health*, December 1995.

Kahn, J., "Homeopathic Remedy Relieves Allergic Asthma Symptoms," *Medical Tribune*, 11, January 5, 1995.

Panos, M. B., Heimlich, J., *Homeopathic Medicine at Home*, G.P. Putnam's Sons, New York., 1980.

Reilly, D. et al, "Is Evidence for Homeopathy Reproducible?" *The Lancet*, 344:1601-1606, December 10, 1994.

"Homeopathy Scores Again," *Townsend Letter for Doctors & Patients*, p.27, June 1996.

Ullman, D., *The Consumer's Guide to Homeopathy*, G.P. Putnam's Sons, New York, 1995.

Hill, N., et al, "A Placebo Controlled Clinical Trial Investigating the Efficacy of a Homeopathic After-Bite Gel in Reducing Mosquito Bite Induced Erythema," *European Journal of Clinical Pharmacology*, 49:103-108, 1995.

INDEX

Cerebrovascular accident,
definition of, 163
Chamomile
for bathing, 78
effectiveness of, 15
Chamomilla, homeopathic
remedy, 294, 295, 306, 317,
319, 321, 324, 332, 333, 334
Chartreuse, 70-71
Chasteberry (*Vitex agnus castus*),
healing herb, 46
Chelation
process, 163, 187, 251
therapy, 248-249
Chelidonium, homeopathic
remedy, 294, 296, 326
Chemical allergies, homeopathic
remedies for, 317
Chemical fertilizers, 189-190
Chicken pox, homeopathic
remedies for, 320
Children
herbal remedies for, 71
homeopathic remedies for,
319-324
lead poisoning of, 244-245
vitamin plan for, 142-143
China Officinalis, homeopathic
remedy, 293-296, 306, 317, 318,
321-323, 325, 326, 329, 332,
333
Chinese herbal tradition, 7, 16, 18
healing herbs, 31, 34, 37, 38, 39-
40, 42, 43, 44, 47, 51, 128
Chinese Medicine Doctors, 86
Chloride, essential element, 178
Chlorine, 126, 195
Cholesterol, 171
definition of, 163, 251
reduction of, 82, 96, 101
types of, 166, 167
Cholestyramine, 209
Choline, supplement, 100, 101
Chromium (trace mineral), 105,
107, 175, 178, 182, 191, 200,
221-224

dietary sources of, 217, 224
Chromium picolinate, 222-224
Chronic, definition of, 163
Chymotrypsin, enzyme, 131, 133
Cicuta, homeopathic remedy, 315
Cimicifuga, homeopathic remedy,
295, 334
Cinchona bark, 16, 263
Circulation, herbs for, 82
Citrulline, amino acid, 113
Clematis, homeopathic remedy,
319
Cleopatra, 7, 27
"Clinical picture," 274, 285
Clovers, for bathing, 78
Cobalamin, 95, 98-99
Cobalt (trace mineral) 105, 107,
177, 178, 181, 182, 221, 224
dietary sources of, 217, 224
interactions, 216
Cocculus Indicus, homeopathic
remedy, 294, 326, 329, 330,
332, 333
Codeine, 45
Coenzymes, 132-133
definition of, 163, 251
Coenzyme Q10 (CoQ10), antioxidant, 126-127
Coffee, homeopathic remedy,
295, 317, 324, 325, 331
Colchicum, homeopathic remedy,
294-295
Colds
herbal first aid kit, 59
homeopathic remedies for, 330
for children, 320
relief from, 70, 73-74, 82
Colic
homeopathic remedies for,
319-320
relief from, 65, 67
Collagen, 181-182, 225
definition of, 163, 251-252
"Colloid" suspensions, 183
Colocynthis, homeopathic
remedy, 317, 320, 329, 333